THE HOSPITAL RESEARCH AND EDUCATIONAL TRUST
An Affiliate of the American Hospital Association

Management of Rural Primary Care— Concepts and Cases

Edited by Gerald E. Bisbee Jr.

With support from the W. K. Kellogg Foundation

Designer and Illustrator: Patricia Job
Compositor: Black Dot
Printer: Pioneer Press Inc.

Library of Congress Cataloging in Publication Data

Main entry under title:

Management of rural primary care.

   1. Rural health services—Administration.
2. Clinics, Rural—Administration.   3. Rural health
services—Case studies.   I. Bisbee, Gerald E.
II. Hospital Research and Educational Trust.
[DNLM: 1. Primary health care—Organ.   2. Rural
health.   3. Community health centers—Organ.
WA 390 M266]
RA771.M26   362.1'0425   81-13296
ISBN 0-87914-057-7   AACR2

Trust Catalog Number: 567080

In 1976, the W.K. Kellogg Foundation awarded $3.5 million to the Hospital Research and Educational Trust to administer the Innovations in Ambulatory Primary Care demonstration project. *Kathleen L. Murrin* directed the project over its entire life and worked with more than 20 primary care delivery programs in predominately rural areas of medical underservice. The success of their primary care delivery efforts and of the overall project has been due in large part to Ms. Murrin's devotion and expert guidance. Her conceptual framework and her documentation during the project provided the foundation and many of the insights for the development of this book.

Several other staff of the Hospital Research and Educational Trust made significant contributions to this book and the project on which it was based. They are: *Christine P. Howell,* who was principal author of the case studies and managed the editorial and production processes for the book; *Kathy S. Kohn,* group director for the Hospital Research and Educational Trust and reviewer and advisor for the book; and *Rosemary L. Summers,* who was coordinator for the book and contributing author of the case studies.

Contents

Concepts

Cases

Christine P. Howell
Rosemary L. Summers

Foreword

This book is designed essentially to guide current and future managers and practitioners in the organization, management and operation of ambulatory primary care centers. For many years, people in rural communities have faced serious difficulties obtaining primary health care. This concern, shared by both the public and the providers of health services, led to a variety of solution-seeking actions in the mid-1970s. Several private philanthropies, among them the W.K. Kellogg Foundation, supported demonstration projects to improve access to and availability of health care for rural areas, to address the quality of service and to strengthen the management of rural ambulatory health care organizations. At the same time, a number of important pieces of federal legislation were passed. They included new methods for financing and reimbursing ambulatory health care and increasing the supply of physicians in areas with physician shortages.

The effect of these efforts and others has been to ameliorate the scarcity of critical health services for many rural Americans. New and creative models for ambulatory primary care have emerged, and effective substitution of appropriate ambulatory services for inpatient hospital care has been demonstrated. Finally, the development of ambulatory care networks by organizations such as community hospitals, medical centers, group practices, foundations for medical care and other established community health agencies has helped these organizations become more responsive to the communities they serve.

The W.K. Kellogg Foundation supported the development and dissemination of this book in order to document and share the experiences of the Innovations in Ambulatory Primary Care project and the valuable information and insight of present-day experts in the field of ambulatory primary care. As rural primary care organizations emerged in the 1970s, so did issues associated with their organizational design, financial and human resources, and planning and viability.

Accompanying the conceptual approaches to organization, management and operation of primary care practices presented in the articles are the real-life experiences of eight health centers that participated in the Innovations in Ambulatory Primary Care project. Their successes and problems in center development and operations are intended to give readers the opportunity to apply critical analytic and problem-solving skills necessary in the rural primary care environment.

It is the hope of the W.K. Kellogg Foundation that family

physicians, group practice managers, rural health care leaders, hospital administrators working in shortage-area communities, physician extenders, community leaders in small cities and towns, and future practitioners and their teachers who are seeking to improve health care for the American public will benefit from what has been learned through these real-life demonstrations.

The Foundation is pleased to have supported this major endeavor in ambulatory primary care and the development of this important educational resource.

Robert A. DeVries
Program Director
W.K. Kellogg Foundation
Battle Creek, Michigan

Acknowledgements

This book could not have been developed without the support and involvement of many people beyond the contributors cited specifically. The following individuals and groups deserve recognition and appreciation for helping to make this publication a reality:

☐ The IAPC primary care centers that agreed to participate in case studies, including the communities, the sponsors and the center staff who were willing to be scrutinized for the benefit of those who might learn from their experiences.

☐ All who reviewed the manuscript or parts of it, especially Roy Penchansky of the University of Michigan; Mary Alice Krill of the Center for Research in Ambulatory Health Care Administration; and Eugenia Shuller of the American College of Hospital Administrators.

☐ Caryl Carpenter for pretesting several of the case studies with her students.

☐ The IAPC steering committee members for their guidance and support in both the project and the book's development: Odin W. Anderson, Ph.D., professor and director, University of Chicago; Colin W. Churchill; Lawrence A. Hill, president, Health Facilities Management Group, Houston; and Charles E. Morrill, M.D., director, Grand Rapids Family Practice Residency, St. Mary's Hospital.

☐ Numerous Trust staff members and freelance editors, including Patricia Robertson, who typed and retyped manuscript and performed countless other tasks for the book; Helen Strand, who was part of the original research team for the book; Michael Carbine, Cynthia DeWitt, Kathi Esqueda, Maureen Flanagan, Margaret Peisert, Dianne Spenner and Tracy Torres, who assisted in editing and proofreading; and Anita Cooper and Karin Dawkins, who provided clerical support.

Introduction

The Innovations in Ambulatory Primary Care demonstration project funded by the W.K. Kellogg Foundation had two major objectives: to foster new models of locally-initiated primary care services in underserved areas; and to identify, address and document the organizational, financial and management issues that were expected to surface in a small, rural ambulatory primary care center. By monitoring the primary care centers during their early years, the project was able to, first, identify the major factors that influenced the initiation and continuation of center operations and, second, provide assistance and guidance to the centers and their sponsors in addressing those factors.

The Kellogg Foundation and the Hospital Research and Educational Trust, administrator of the IAPC project, wanted others to have the opportunity to learn from the knowledge gained and the experiences of the project. It was not the intent, however, to merely describe the project; rather, the intent was to produce a resource that would help others apply the experiences and lessons of the project to the range of organizational, management and financial variables that exist in the delivery of rural primary care services.

With that premise in mind, this book was designed to (1) present the major factors influencing the initiation and continuation of a rural primary care center, (2) convey the interrelated and interdependent nature of those factors and (3) provide an opportunity to apply that body of knowledge to the study of actual situations and the resolution of actual problems faced by rural primary care centers. The audiences for whom this book is intended include: undergraduate, graduate and continuing education students and faculty in hospital administration, health planning and primary care residency programs; managers, practitioners and planners of primary care practice organizations; and the management staffs of hospitals, public health departments and other organizations involved in or contemplating rural primary care services delivery.

This book contains two sections: (1) articles that discuss the issues, concepts and practices applicable to the organization and management of rural primary care centers and (2) case studies based on the IAPC project that translate those concepts into actual management and organizational situations.

Articles

The five articles were developed specifically for this volume by professionals with a wide range of knowledge and experience in primary care theory and practice. These chapters provide managers and planners with a conceptual basis for effective decision making in response to the major issues facing the rural primary care field today.

The historical perspective of the medical care system's impact on rural primary care can provide a basis for understanding the issues facing health care professionals in rural areas today. The first chapter, "Laying the Groundwork: Issues Facing Rural Primary Care," by Kathleen L. Murrin, was developed with this in mind. The chapter also documents IAPC project findings, particularly as they substantiate material presented in the other articles and in the case study situations.

In the book's second chapter, "Organizational Design and the Management of Primary Care Services," Arnold D. Kaluzny and Thomas R. Konrad present four basic models of organizational design for the delivery of primary care in rural areas and relate alternative management strategies to each design.

Caryl E. Carpenter, in "Human Resources Planning and Management," discusses human resource issues vital to all primary care practices—recruitment, retention, performance effectiveness, alternative provider models and management practices relating to human resource development and utilization.

Financing of rural primary care is a complex activity that can entangle centers in confusing and conflicting priorities. The chapter "Financing the Development of Rural Primary Care Centers," by Roland Palmer and Ann Eward, presents a framework for developing a financial resource strategy in an ambulatory primary care organization.

The final chapter in the first section of the book was developed in recognition of the relationship between short-term operational requirements and longer term planning and strategies. In "Managing the Future through Planned Organizational Change," Stephen F. Loebs, Judy Johnson and Rosemary L. Summers discuss the major factors that influence the long-range viability of any health center and provide insight to the crucial issue of achieving financial viability and self-sufficiency.

Case Studies

The second section of the book consists of eight case studies that are designed to bridge the gap between concepts and practice. The field of management education has found that study of the experiences of other managers can be valuable in developing the skills necessary for effective administrative action.

The eight IAPC project sites selected for case study development were no more or less successful than any of the other project sites. The selection was based solely on clarity of the issues chosen for illustration, geographic location and organizational model of the site.

Intensive on-site interviews with many individuals at each of the eight sites, as well as extensive supporting documentation from the sites and sponsors, formed the basis for the case studies in this book. Each case study was subjected to an in-depth review process. Three of the cases were pretested with first- or second-year health administration students. Each of the sites reviewed the case study and agreed to its publication. *As a courtesy to the centers and people who participated in this process, all of the cases have been disguised and somewhat fictionalized to protect the identities of people and places.* It should be remembered, however, that the case studies are based on real situations.

The case studies are not a narration of events with a beginning and an end. They were written to develop analytical and problem-solving skills related to organizing, managing, financing and operating a primary care center. Actual situations confronting administrators are rarely manifested in a single, isolated problem. Similarly, each case study contains overlapping management and/or organizational issues. Each case, however, has a major emphasis. The case studies were designed so that the reader or student can identify and analyze the overlapping problems of each case and develop an appropriate plan for problem resolution.

Gerald E. Bisbee Jr., Ph.D., Editor
Vice President and Director,
The Hospital Research and Educational Trust

Concepts

1
Laying the Groundwork: Issues Facing Rural Primary Care

Kathleen L. Murrin, M.A.

Ms. Murrin was project director of the Innovations in Ambulatory Primary Care project, the Hospital Research and Educational Trust, Chicago.

Laying the Groundwork: Issues Facing Rural Primary Care

More than 26 million of the 66 million rural Americans are medically underserved (Lichty and Zuvekas, 1980). Despite the fact that the term "medical underservice" has not been defined explicitly since its inception in the 1970s, this term and related measures were used extensively in health planning and health policy development and implementation during the past decade (Kane and others, 1979). There was a high level of national concern during the 1970s over the decline of rural health care resources, a concern that went beyond the inadequacies of definitions and numbers.

During the 1970s, millions of dollars in grant funding were focused on the plight of rural health care delivery and the condition of medical underservice in rural areas. Major funding initiatives in both the public and private sectors addressed the issue of access to services, concentrating on the availability or shortage of human resources. A major focus of these initiatives was the development of community-based medical practices or primary health care centers as alternatives to the disappearing country doctor's office. Their intent was to improve access to services in rural communities by enhancing provider recruitment and retention and by responding to identified community health care needs.

Forces in the larger health care arena influenced the rural health care delivery initiatives and funding of the 1970s. As health care costs soared in the late 1960s (after the introduction of Medicare and Medicaid), the federal government began seeking more cost-effective methods for the delivery of services. The resultant increased regulatory activity in the early 1970s prompted health care institutions to look for new products as substitutes for costly inpatient care and for new markets. Ambulatory and primary care were viewed as a potential product substitute, while the growing social concern over the declining physician population of small towns and rural areas generated a new market potential. These factors, combined with the timely availability of demonstration grant funding and other equivalents of risk venture funds, provided the impetus for concerted efforts to develop rural primary care health centers.

Although the outcomes of the rural initiatives of the late 1970s are only now unfolding, there is much to be learned from this intense period of demonstration in terms of both the achievements and the problems experienced by the rural health center demonstration sites and their sponsors. In the years ahead, the continuing experiences of those models will further document whether the initiatives of the 1970s have promoted beneficial systemwide change.

Following a definition of terms related to rural primary care, this chapter presents an overview of the major historical events in the U.S. health care system, emphasizing the major funding initiatives and policy developments of the 1960s and 1970s in response to the problem of rural medical underservice. With that broad background, the chapter examines the Innovations in Ambulatory Primary Care (IAPC) project funded by the W. K. Kellogg Foundation, identifying findings and observations to date and what those findings and observations (as well as other initiatives undertaken during the 1970s) indicate for the operation of rural primary care centers. The final section of the chapter presents conclusions about rural primary care delivery assimilated from experience to date.

Definition of Terms

Primary care is basic sick and well-maintenance care provided to patients when they first contact a health care provider. Organizationally, it is the entry point to the health care system, which itself is subdivided into three functional levels—primary, secondary and tertiary. Primary care constitutes 85 to 90 percent of all medical diagnosis and treatment and is most often provided in the physician's office. Secondary care entails services of a specialist nature provided either in an ambulatory (office or clinic) setting or in the inpatient setting of a community hospital. Tertiary care refers to the highly complex and sophisticated services of subspecialists typically available through a medical center (Parker, 1974).

Primary care is not synonymous with ambulatory care. Ambulatory care refers to any health care service provided when individuals are not admitted to a bed in a hospital or a health care institution (Goldsmith, 1977). Ambulatory care encompasses a range of services from primary care through specialty, subspecialty, multidisciplinary and high-technology services. Ambulatory care became the generic terminology for the full range of noninpatient services provided by health care institutions. (Even though physician's offices have long been in the business of ambulatory care, the terminology was not typically applied there.) In its earliest use, the term ambulatory primary care differentiated hospital-sponsored primary care services from hospital-sponsored specialty and subspecialty outpatient clinics.

Ambulatory primary care now refers to primary care services delivered in an organized setting; that is, a medical practice with an identity independent from that of the particular individual physician(s) working in the practice (Jonas and Rimer, 1977). This distinction is not always apparent to the individual consumer, and ambulatory primary care continues to be identified with the individual physician. This is particularly true in rural towns, where consumers often expect that primary care services will be delivered by their personal private physician on a continuous basis. Rural consumers also tend to expect not only the same coping and caring qualities attributed to country physicians of the past, but also the vastly improved curing capacity of the modern physician. However, in a century-long quest for cure and subspecialty technology, the medical profession and its attendant health care system and educational process have become more and more removed from these care demands of the general public, although this disengagement occurred more slowly in rural areas. As rural general practitioners moved toward retirement, the priorities established by medical education and the health care system did not allow for or encourage their replacement, nor attempt to address changing consumer expectations.

While the term "rural" implies a sparse geographic dispersion of a relatively small number of people, it is still an arbitrary term. Two frequently used definitions are: the population residing in the open country and in communities of less than 2,500; and the population located in a county outside a Standard Metropolitan Statistical Area (Madison and Bernstein, 1976).

A more practical definition would include trade center communities of 2,500 to 10,000 upon which many rural residents depend. As more of their services and economic functions are assumed by larger cities, these trade centers have less in common with larger cities and increasingly resemble their surrounding small villages and rural areas (Copp, 1976).

Rural is not a homogeneous classification. Geographically, it comprises areas that are remote and isolated as well as communities that border major SMSAs. There also are wide variations in the nature of people and occupations in these communities, among them farming, mining, fishing, small industry and recreational enterprises. Underlying the demographic variations, however, are some shared expectations and attitudes that have led to a distinctly rural impression of life that affects business practices and patterns of seeking health care.

Rural areas typically are characterized by a low population concentration, relative lack of wealth (with the exception of some rich farm areas), a disproportionately high share of elderly as younger people leave rural areas, a short supply of services in general and a lower level of education. Talent and youth have tended to leave rural areas, resulting in a scarcity of trained leadership talent (Madison and Bernstein, 1976). Contributing to this leadership drain is the limited availability of organizational bases, making it difficult to obtain resources and attract talent. Rural "institutions" (schools, general stores, general medical practitioners, citizen governments and churches or preachers) have aged or declined in number as transportation enhanced the availability of similar services in other communities. This trend began to reverse in the 1970s with the first hint of a return migration to small towns and rural areas and population growth in the sunbelt states.

Historical Overview: 1900-1959

During the first half of this century, the U.S. population increased from under 90 million to 150 million. Approximately 60 percent of the 90 million people in 1900 lived in rural areas; by 1950, only 35 percent of the population lived in these areas. The forces of industrialization and urbanization, together with modern transportation, drained rural areas of two of their natural resources: land and youth. In a very real sense, much of rural America became a casualty of the industrial revolution (Mott and Roemer, 1948).

American medical education, on the other hand, was a beneficiary of this period. Medicine became one of the chief recipients of both the growing philanthropic benevolence of the urban wealthy and the scientific knowledge and technological advances of industrial progress. Philanthropic foundations enabled private medical schools to make the improvements suggested by the 1910 Flexner report on medical education and to implement advances in technical skills, equipment and medical knowledge (Stevens, 1971). Both the Flexner report recommendations and the resources of urban philanthropists served to establish medicine as a largely urban enterprise and to standardize the medical education of general physicians at urban facilities. In 1910, the Flexner report dealt with the gap between what was then known about medicine as science and what was being taught in substandard medical schools. Fifty years later, the gap was between what was being taught at medical schools of the highest standard and what was needed to alleviate the medical underservice of a great portion of the American population (Geyman, 1979).

Medicine began to differentiate into medical specialties as general medical education became standardized and as technology began to play an increasingly important role in medicine. The emergence of surgery and the concomitant advances and reforms in medical education stimulated hospital development. Once again, urban wealth and social concern were channeled into medicine, specifically the hospital movement. The approximately 200 hospitals that existed around the turn of the century typically were large in size, were operated as charitable institutions under the auspices of ethnic or religious groups and were located in a few major cities. By 1927, there were 6,807 hospitals, 4,322 of which were general hospitals (Corwin, 1946).

Before the Flexner report, medicine was being practiced by erratically trained or apprenticed solo general practitioners. The professional elitism of specialty medical training stimulated by the Flexner report ignored the majority of these existing physicians, most of whom were general practitioners located in rural areas, and concentrated on physicians in training, most of whom would locate in urban areas.

Schematically, the health service "system" in this country first resembled a series of unconnected dots (representing physicians) scattered across the surface of a map, with concentrations in the major cities. During the 1930s, this uncoordinated system of general practitioners began to be replaced by an uncoordinated system of specialists, with growing concentrations in the major cities (Stevens, 1971). Questions of coordination and distribution of services were becoming more acute each year.

The critical financial situation and social turbulence of the Depression focused national attention on the rising costs of medical care at the very time the population was experiencing an increasing inability to pay for services. The Depression brought the federal government into health services, although government involvement at this time was limited to the financially destitute and consisted of efforts such as the categorical grants-in-aid programs of the Social Security Act of 1935 and the Farm Security Administration of the U.S. Deparment of Agriculture.

The Farm Security Administration (FSA), directed toward meeting medical services needs among low-income and economically marginal farm families, was an important first step in rural primary care. The FSA developed a federally subsidized, prepaid medical program that, by its peak in 1942, was providing for 600,000 people in 1,100 rural counties and an additional 150,000 people under its migratory farm worker sector (Roemer, 1976). The program declined after World War II when federal assistance was withdrawn.

Another legacy of the Depression was the deteriorating financial situation of voluntary hospitals. The number of new hospitals declined during the Depression and World War II years, and between 1940 and 1944 few if any hospitals were built or reconstructed except in selected war-production areas and within the federal hospital system.

The Depression also stimulated the development of health insurance programs, and the rapid growth of the nonprofit Blue Cross and Blue Shield insurance plans during the 1940s contributed significantly to stabilizing the financial picture for existing hospitals. The growth in insurance was stimulated by collective bargaining for fringe benefits in the workplace during the wage-controlled war years and the post-World War II era.

The health insurance movement had little impact on rural health care delivery and rural populations. Individual farm families and people living in rural trade centers were not as easily enrolled as were the employee groups of urban industries. Even when rural people were insured, it was more often under the individual enrollment type of indemnity policy sold by commercial carriers—policies that tended to have higher premiums and fewer benefits. Thus, while about 75 percent of the population in all occupations had some form of insurance protection (usually hospitalization) in 1970, only 37 percent of farm laborers and foremen had this protection. Moreover, relatively few rural residents received sick pay or other income maintenance benefits (Lane, 1976).

After World War II, the health care role of the federal government entered a new phase. Through the Hospital Survey and Construction Act of 1946 (PL 70-725), commonly referred to as the Hill-Burton program, the federal government invested heavily in the construction and modernization of nonfederal health care facilities (more than $3.7 billion between 1947 and 1971). Assisting in 30 percent of all hospital construction projects between 1947 and 1962, the government played an important role in the survival and revival of the nonprofit community hospital. This program marked the beginning of significant governmental interaction with the private health care delivery system. It also represented an early attempt at areawide planning and regionalization by requiring that master plans for health care facility needs be developed in each state (Clarke, 1980).

It was not until Hill-Burton and its required statewide master plans that much attention was directed to the medical resource capabilities of rural areas. The Hill-Burton program was established with a rural priority in its mission. Nearly 40 percent of all projects undertaken during its existence were related to communities of under 10,000 population, and two-thirds of all Hill-Burton-financed general hospital beds were built in smaller cities, towns or rural areas (McNerney and Reidel, 1962).

Historically, quite unlike their urban counterparts, rural hospitals were small and typically were proprietary hospitals operated by physician owners. The number of proprietary hospitals in rural America grew markedly during the first quarter of the 20th century. These hospitals frequently were converted residences with six or seven patient beds and living quarters for the doctor's family on a separate floor. Health care delivery, as well as decision making about rural health care resources, was the responsibility of these rural general practitioners.

Many of the events that took place in urban areas in the first half of the century—among them the advances and sophistication in medical technology and education, the population migration, the health insurance movement and philanthropy—left most rural hospitals throughout America substantially behind in the ability to provide quality inpatient care. The U.S. Census Bureau counted 3,539 proprietary hospital facilities in 1940 that were not recognized or included by the American Medical Association in its registration of 6,201 U.S. hospitals (Corwin, 1946). Hill-Burton assistance, because it was limited to public or voluntary nonprofit facilities, contributed significantly to the decline and/or closure of many of these small, proprietary, rural hospitals. At the same time, Hill-Burton so improved the quantity and quality of rural nonproprietary hospital resources that it largely eliminated the bed-supply disparity between predominantly rural and urban states. One goal of Hill-Burton had been to enhance physician recruitment to rural areas by increasing the availability of hospital facilities. However, the impact of Hill-Burton on physician distribution in rural areas was considerably less dramatic than it was on rural bed numbers.

Another early approach to redistributing physicians was the Commonwealth Fund's medical student fellowship program during the 1930s, which included a rural service obligation. Despite discouraging retention rates, several state governments launched similar programs during the 1940s.

During the 1950s, the Sears Roebuck Foundation introduced its

Community Medical Assistance Program (CMAP) to assist rural communities in building medical clinic facilities. This program was based on the assumption, similar to Hill-Burton's, that modern facilities would enhance physician recruitment to rural areas. Between 1957 and 1970, the CMAP provided design, fund-raising and planning assistance to 165 rural physician offices. Several years later, 132 of these 165 offices (80 percent) had at least one physician working in the office/clinic. However, the turnover rate was high—30 percent of the physicians remained for one year or less (Kane and others, 1975). This program demonstrated that, while a new facility was helpful in recruiting physicians, it did not ensure their retention. And while CMAP relied heavily on strong community motivation and commitment, it did not address the modern physician's growing concerns over long hours and heavy work loads, professional and cultural isolation and income potential during the start-up of a new medical practice.

Another significant rural program during the 1950s was the United Mine Workers of America (UMWA) Welfare and Retirement Fund, an innovative fringe benefit won at the bargaining table that provided for a full range of health services benefits for miners and their families. These services eventually included a series of prepaid physician group practice clinics run by consumer boards representing the local communities and a regional chain of 10 nonprofit hospitals with provision for numerous outpatient services. Financial difficulties beset the fund when the bottom fell out of the coal industry in the early 1960s, but it had a significant impact on the medical care delivery system in southern Appalachia (Berney, 1978).

Rural Primary Care Efforts: 1960-1980

Several factors contributed to the increasing importance of medical care delivery as a national priority during the 1960s and 1970s. Health care was increasingly viewed as a "right" rather than a privilege. Public expectations about medical care and social services in general were rising. Health care consumers were becoming better informed, more demanding and more involved in the issues of availability, accessibility and fragmentation of health services, particularly as they related to the disappearance or decline of their own personal physicians. The health care field, previously a loose aggregation of social service endeavors, had become an $80-billion industry that accounted for 7.6 percent of the gross national product (Falk, 1972).

While government programs initiated in the mid-1960s continued to foster facilities, education and medical research, they shifted attention to the financing mechanisms and organizational arrangements that appeared to control access to these resources. By the end of the 1960s, the federal government was heavily involved in the private sector of medicine. American hospitals were flourishing and modern medicine had made tremendous strides in specialty fields and medical technology. There was a growing identification of and concern over issues of scarcity of facilities and personnel, overspecialization of medical providers and rising costs. Consumers were becoming increasingly disturbed by the social and personal implications of these issues.

The 1965 Social Security amendments were intended to eliminate economic barriers to using the traditional medical care system for the elderly and disabled (Title XVIII, Medicare) and the poor (Title XIX, Medicaid). However, the medically underserved rural population represented a significant gap in the programs' intent. Both Medicare and Medicaid discriminated against rural communities through lower reimbursement levels for the same kinds of services provided in urban areas with higher prevailing charges (Kane and others, 1978). The differences were sufficiently large that a reversal of funds—from rural to urban areas—occurred. This "cross-subsidization" amounted to almost $300 million in fiscal year 1975 for the Medicare Part B program alone (Ricketts and others, 1979). In addition, many rural physicians would not accept Medicare assignment because of the government involvement and the required paper work. Thus, for many rural people, entitlement to services through Medicare and Medicaid only accented the scarcity of physicians and the lack of mechanisms from which to secure services.

A declining number of physicians in rural areas was another result of the national migration trend and the concentration of technology and specialization in the major cities. While the total number of physicians in direct patient care increased from 119 per 100,000 population in 1950 to 137 in 1970, there were only 41 physicians per 100,000 population in the most rural areas in 1970 versus 192 per 100,000 population in the most urban counties. Significantly for rural areas, the overall number of general practitioners declined by one-half between 1930 and 1970 (Coleman, 1976).

The rural general practitioners who remained in general practice tended to be older than their urban counterparts, had limited practices and were retiring from practice and dying at a faster rate than were urban physicians. They also were not, for the most part, being replaced by new physicians. At the same time, health level comparisons indicated more chronic illness, more days lost from work and higher death rates from accidents in rural areas. In addition, rural areas, along with the rest of the nation, were affected by providers' increasing focus on episodic care of acute illnesses, which contributed to fragmentation and lack of coordination of health care services.

Three major national reports published in 1966 (the Millis, Willard and Folsom reports) prompted the medical profession to address the problems of overspecialization and fragmentation. In 1969, the medical specialty of family practice was established, emphasizing the generalist role in medicine, the family as the unit of care, comprehensiveness and continuity of care and ready access to care (Geyman, 1978).

Coinciding with the medical profession's response to overspecialization and fragmentation was the government's attention to the maldistribution of providers. Health manpower legislation introduced during the 1970s was specifically directed toward the predominantly rural problems of maldistribution of health personnel by specialty and location, inadequate numbers of primary care practitioners and health administrators, excessive numbers of inadequately trained foreign medical graduates and health personnel whose professional capabilities had become outdated.

The Emergency Health Personnel Act of 1970 (PL 91-623) created the National Health Service Corps (NHSC), a federal program to provide health care personnel to areas experiencing a shortage. The Health Professions Educational Assistance Act of 1976 (PL 94-484) reestablished the NHSC and augmented the 1972 Public Health and NHSC Scholarship Training Program, under which loans to medical students could be repaid through clinical service in a designated shortage area. This national program coincided with increasing federal financial incentives (mostly through capitation grants that replaced earlier institutional grants) for medical schools to enroll and graduate students in the primary care specialties of internal medicine, pediatrics and family medicine (Rosenblatt and Moscovice, 1980).

During the late 1960s, neighborhood health centers were established under a demonstration project of the newly-created Office of Economic Opportunity (OEO). The strategy of this project was to meet health care needs of specific indigent and low-income populations through a multidisciplinary team approach to health care delivery and community involvement in both policymaking and facility operations. By 1973, the 40 existing OEO neighborhood health centers had been transferred to the aegis of the HEW Bureau of

Community Health Services. Twelve of these centers were in rural areas, twenty-six in urban areas and two in urban-rural areas (Lewis and others, 1976).

The late 1960s through the 1970s also was a period of considerable health planning and medical resource regionalization activity. Federal grants for regional medical programs were intended to geographically disperse medical knowledge, traditionally centered in urban universities, to outlying areas. These were followed by Area Health Education Centers, designed to provide continuing education for health personnel in areas outside the urban university setting. Health planning legislation was intended, among other things, to expand consumer participation in health planning and achieve a more balanced geographic distribution of health resources.

During the 1970s, several local and state efforts, including the Office of Rural Health Services in North Carolina and the Kentucky Health Development Association, attempted to improve the availability of health care services and providers in rural areas. In 1975 and 1976, federally- and privately-funded initiatives at a national level attempted to enhance the recruitment of providers to rural areas by creating rural medical practice organizations with an environment that would foster long-term retention of providers.

Federal attempts to foster rural practice organizations included the Health Underserved Rural Areas (HURA) and Rural Health Initiative (RHI) programs, inaugurated within a year of each other and combined a year later (in 1976) under HEW's Bureau of Community Health Services. The HURA program emphasized research and evaluation of existing models of health care delivery (in 1979 it was succeeded by the Primary Care Research and Demonstration program), while RHI was an effort to more effectively direct federal resources toward the development of comprehensive primary care delivery systems in medically underserved rural areas. The first step in this program was to fund and establish rural primary care practice organizations as demonstration sites. These sites relied to a considerable degree on the placement of health professionals through the NHSC, which in turn emphasized the placement of assignees in community-supported practices. All three programs—HURA, RHI and NHSC—represented a joint venture between the federal government and local communities.

Two privately-funded national demonstration programs introduced in 1975 and 1976 were the Innovations in Ambulatory Primary Care project, funded by the W.K. Kellogg Foundation and developed and administered by the Hospital Research and Educational

Trust, and the Rural Community Practice Models Program (or Rural Practice Project) funded by the Robert Wood Johnson Foundation and administered through the University of North Carolina School of Medicine.

These federal and private demonstration programs in rural primary care shared five characteristics:

☐ They attempted to improve access to and the quality of health service delivery in rural areas of medical underservice.

☐ They attempted to enhance the attractiveness of rural areas with respect to recruitment and retention of health personnel, especially physicians, through the development of financially stable medical practice organizations.

☐ They attempted to provide for the comprehensive needs of the patient by coordinating and integrating service delivery with other local or categorical community services, as well as with hospital and specialty services.

☐ They strongly supported the use of nonphysician providers and emphasized community involvement, education and leadership.

☐ The medical practice sites were to become financially self-sufficient after grant funding expired.

These federal and foundation initiatives provided millions of dollars over a five-year period (1975 to 1980) for the establishment of medical practice organizations/primary care centers within rural communities. At the same time, the federal government initiated two efforts to improve the availability of capital and reimbursement monies for these sites. In 1977, the Rural Health Clinic Services Act (PL 95-210) allowed cost-related Medicare reimbursement for nurse practitioner and physician assistant services provided by health centers in rural federally-designated medically underserved areas. In 1978, HEW entered into an agreement with the Farmer's Home Administration (Department of Agriculture) under which rural health centers supported by RHI funding could acquire low-interest loans for facility construction.

Starting in 1978, a comprehensive evaluation of rural primary care initiatives was undertaken by the Health Services Research Center at the University of North Carolina. The project was funded by the Robert Wood Johnson Foundation in coordination with the Office of the Assistant Secretary for Planning and Evaluation/Health of the Department of Health and Human Services. To date, this evaluation has identified over 650 philanthropically or publicly supported rural practice organizations established primarily during the 1970s. The purpose of the evaluation is to compare various forms of rural primary care organizations operating in a broad range of community environments. Outcomes being assessed include access to care, patient and provider satisfaction and stability of the organization—both in terms of provider recruitment and retention and fiscal viability. This evaluation is due to be completed in 1982 (Schonfeld and others, 1981).

Innovations in Ambulatory Primary Care Project

In March 1976, the W.K. Kellogg Foundation awarded the Hospital Research and Educational Trust (the Trust) a $3.5-million grant to demonstrate innovative approaches to the delivery of ambulatory primary care in medically underserved areas, primarily underserved rural areas. The Kellogg Foundation and the Trust wanted to establish a variety of models for delivering primary care that would address the major issue of access to medical care. The Foundation was particularly interested in funding and evaluating a diversity of organizational models to provide alternative approaches to problems of medical underservice.

The Innovations in Ambulatory Primary Care (IAPC) project sought to make maximum use of existing organizations and attempted to increase the sensitivity and responsiveness of organizations to community health care needs. It was felt that this strategy would direct available resources to underserved communities while linking these communities with their own incipient care systems. The strategy also would shift some responsibility for health and medical care from the solo physician to the community and existing organizations.

In early 1977, demonstration grants were awarded to 23 organizations representing a broad spectrum of organizational sponsorship, geographic characteristics and provider diversity. Grantees included nine hospitals, seven community health care corporations, two universities, two public health departments and three nonprofit provider organizations. Six sites were located in the northeast, three in the southeast, nine in the midwest, three in the northwest and two in the southwest. In terms of provider diversity, there were four nurse practitioner sites, four physician-only sites and fifteen physician/ midlevel practitioner teams.

While 23 grants originally were awarded for a two-year period, funding was withdrawn from three sites after one year. The grants ranged from $84,000 to $195,000 per grantee, and 11 sites requested and received supplemental funding for an additional year. Ultimately, $3 million was spent over three years to assist the development of 20 primary care centers (19 rural and one inner-city).

Grant funding tended to introduce a relatively major risk factor for the sponsors and communities in terms of both fiscal accountability and the need to act quickly within a limited time frame. The very nature of these new developments (risk and quick action) was stressful, especially for those unfamiliar with grant program requirements. Because crises developed almost immediately, technical assistance to the sites became as important as site funding, and most sites needed help in mastering the complexity of the health care system.

All but two of the IAPC primary care centers were located in small towns of less than 5,000 population. These centers typically had one to three medical providers on site and annual budgets ranging from $50,000 to $200,000. All but three of the centers were new endeavors initiated at the time of the grant. The three exceptions were centers that already had been delivering services for two to four years and were awarded funding to stabilize and expand operations.

During the first funding year, 74,000 patient visits were recorded at the 20 sites. These visits represented $2 million in operating expenses, for an average cost of $27 per visit. During the next year, 122,000 patient visits were recorded, representing $3 million in operating expenses, or an average cost of $24.60 per visit. Over 127,000 visits were recorded at the 11 sites funded during the supplemental year, representing just under $2.5 million in operating expenses, or an average cost of less than $20 per visit.

All the IAPC rural initiatives shared a common goal—increased and improved access to care for rural Americans. Although availability is one dimension of access, access involves more than simply locating a health care resource in a community—it is the fit between the resource and the community or clients (Penchansky and Thomas, 1981). Access is an enabling process that begins with a definition of need, includes the community's ability to reach, obtain and afford needed services and continues to the actual utilization of services (Sheps and Bachar, 1978).

At this writing, 19 of the 20 IAPC primary care sites are still in operation even though grant funding expired in 1980. Findings and observations to date about the successes and/or problems associated with the project can be grouped under four areas: provider recruitment and retention; organizational development and stability; financing; and community responsiveness.

Provider Recruitment and Retention

All IAPC sites were able to recruit providers to their communities, although some fared better than others. The IAPC sites strived to provide a professional practice environment and address physician concerns regarding the financial and professional risks of establishing a rural medical practice by providing an appropriate facility, arranging for support staff and office management, assuring physician remuneration and securing back-up coverage for the provider. When IAPC sites experienced provider recruitment problems, they were most often symptomatic of underlying organizational stress and confusion or conflict, either within the sponsoring organization, between the sponsoring organization and the community or both.

Other factors observed to affect physician recruitment and retention were the economic viability of the community and physician attitude toward rural practice. The IAPC sites were not located in the most economically poor sections of the country (the deep South or Appalachia).* The only rural IAPC sites serving a predominantly indigent community or population were the public health department-sponsored sites, and these typically experienced higher turnover in physicians than did other sites during the funding period. Sites that were more remote than rural (typically more than a 40-minute drive to a larger community and more isolated from system resources) encountered greater delays in recruiting providers. Recruiting a physician and establishing a medical practice in town represented, for several IAPC sites, a first step toward improving the local community economy, which in turn enhanced provider recruitment and retention.†

In at least seven of the 20 IAPC sites, a personal characteristic expressed by the recruited providers and shared by their spouses was a strong commitment to a religious or philosophical value system that involved a "missionary spirit" about living in and serving a small rural

---

*In a study of primary care sites by the National Health Service Corps, physician recruitment of Corps assignees was affected by economic status of the community; that is, economic stability had a positive effect on recruitment (Woolf and others, 1981).
†According to Rushing and Wade (1973), community social and economic advantages (and disadvantages) tend to be cumulative, and physician resources are but one part of this cumulative pattern.

community. All of these sites (except for the death of one provider) retained their providers over the three-year funding period.

Conclusive observations about physician retention cannot be drawn, since most IAPC sites have been in existence for less than four years. Because provider retention appears to be correlated with practice growth and stability (Rosenblatt and Moscovice, 1978), and because most practices take several years to move from start-up to an operational growth phase, it is not surprising that physician turnover at the IAPC sites has been relatively high. Despite the problems inherent in starting up, expanding or changing an organization, six of the twenty IAPC sites retained the same physicians through their initial three years of operation.

A study of NHSC assignments showed that one factor positively associated with physician retention was the presence of a hospital or a group practice arrangement, while impediments to retention included service area populations below 4,000 and lack of a hospital or group practice arrangement (Rosenblatt and Moscovice, 1978). Only one IAPC site had a service area population of less than 4,000—a New England site that employed a nurse practitioner (who was still there four years later) with off-site physician coverage. Although only two rural IAPC primary care centers had hospitals in the immediate community, all centers had a strong affiliation with a hospital in the surrounding area. This relationship was viewed as helpful in physician recruitment and retention. Three of the four nurse practitioner sites represented the only solo-provider arrangements (with offsite back-up); half of the IAPC sites had two physicians onsite, and the remainder had a physician/physician extender team.

Organizational Development and Stability: The Practice Environment

Within the variety of IAPC organizational sponsors funded, no single organizational model or sponsor clearly surfaced as more successful or unsuccessful than any other in starting up a rural primary care practice. All sponsors experienced both successes and crises. An important element, however, was how and when successes and problems were identified and in what terms they were defined; it was as important for the center or sponsor to identify successes as it was to account for crises. In the IAPC experience, three factors were observed as influencing organizational development and stability: (1) hospital sponsorship; (2) program management; and (3) the role of the physician.

Hospital Sponsorship

One of the most successful IAPC sites was sponsored by a small rural hospital. However, as the case studies demonstrate, there are inherent conflicts when a hospital, which traditionally has provided inpatient care, begins to provide primary care as well. For the IAPC centers, these conflicts typically were associated with the assignment of both administrative and medical resource priorities by the hospital sponsor. Administrative and medical resources for ambulatory primary care typically were not a high priority of the sponsor. Working with a community group in the primary care setting was an even lower priority, especially when such activities were seen as frustrating and time-consuming by the hospital administration or medical staff.

In the IAPC experience, hospital sponsorship of ambulatory primary care frequently encountered organizational difficulties and reimbursement problems. Of the seven IAPC hospital sponsors, five eventually transferred ownership of the primary care centers either to a community board (particularly if federal funding was involved) or to the physicians for their private practice. One possible reason for this (see Chapter 4) is that hospital ownership of primary care centers may adversely affect hospital reimbursement, particularly for smaller hospitals where the margin for creative accounting is more limited. On the other hand, sponsorship or continuing affiliation can be advantageous to the hospital as well as to the practice organization—for example, through selling needed services to the primary care practice while establishing a referral base for the hospital. Several IAPC hospital sponsors addressed the ownership issue during start-up by assigning the primary care practice to a nonoperating budget account or by funneling funds through a hospital foundation and reaching final decisions about ownership or affiliation later, often at the end of grant funding.

Hospital management frequently could not address the issue of hospital ownership in ways that satisfied the hospital medical staff. Some hospital medical staffs (or, more likely, some influential members of the staff) opposed hospital sponsorship of primary care, particularly when it appeared to be a successful venture. This opposition seemed to arise when the primary care practice was perceived as having a potential competitive edge in its ability to offer services that were more comprehensive than those offered in the offices of the medical staff. These experiences seem to suggest that hospital sponsors should offer similar support services to all physicians on their staff, a position that supports an affiliated rather than an ownership role. This does not negate a sponsorship role for hospitals during start-up. What it likely demonstrates is that a lack of clarity about goals, roles and relationships seriously impedes start-up under any sponsorship, particularly hospital or other institutional sponsorship, where a small, new organization must be integrated with a large, complex, established organization.

Management

The delivery of rural primary care from an organized setting introduced new roles, responsibilities and organizational relationships to the traditional rural office practice. An important ingredient for the effectiveness and efficiency of IAPC primary care practices was the role of the administrator and/or the function of the practice's general management. One skill that appeared to be significant was the capacity to conceptualize corporate purpose and strategy and to invest them with some degree of magnetism. This skill is indispensable for the medical director and/or administrator of a new practice organization and increasingly necessary for the physician in private practice. This skill also is necessary for the community board member involved in managing community development, community board meetings, physician recruitment or board/administrator relationships.

Each IAPC site had at least one charismatic figure who held the program together and kept it moving. Different charismatic individuals emerged during different stages of site development; often during the very early stages it was a founding community board member or provider. Clearly, the vision and the enthusiasm provided by these individuals were necessary elements for success of the practice.

For many IAPC sites, justification for management positions came from the sponsoring organization's increasing awareness of the complexity of organizational development and behavior. Administrators of IAPC sites were either current employees of the sponsoring organization's administration (often an in-kind contribution) or, in the case of community sponsors, were hired by the community board as full- or part-time employees of the practice. In all but one of the 10 institutional-sponsored (hospital or university) IAPC sites, the administrator possessed a master's degree in a health-related field. These administrators were typically young and recent graduates of hospital administration programs. Their incentive for accepting these jobs in rural areas seems to have been the opportunity for greater responsibility at an earlier age than might have been the case in urban health care organizations. In all six community-sponsored IAPC sites, the administrators tended to be older, and their educational background and professional experience were outside the health field.

As was the case in the Rural Practice Project funded by the Robert Wood Johnson Foundation, administrators at IAPC sites typically reported that, despite their backgrounds, they found themselves in unfamiliar territory as they started to develop the new practice model. They lacked experience and practical knowledge about starting up and running a small health care delivery business. There were no "how-to" manuals and few successful models to provide guidance and answers, and success seemed to hinge on the dynamics of the particular community.

A critical success factor for IAPC administrators was the ability to define problems in both organizational and interpersonal terms. Personality conflicts or personal ego struggles at IAPC sites often masked organizational issues or organizational stress. Because these developing organizations were small, personal relationships tended to be more prominent than organizational relationships or dynamics. In addition, the center organizations were new, and the people involved (particularly the community board members) were in new roles. The inexperience and insecurity typical of individuals in new roles exacerbated the already prominent personality issues that arise in small organizations.

Part of the administrator's role is that of intermediary, and at times this involved being the bearer of bad news. It was important to site development that the administrator recognized this role and acted with sensitivity and strength when dealing with the governing or advisory board, the funding agency, providers or the institutional sponsor. Maintaining organizational and functional integrity required a strong commitment on the part of the administrator to confront issues and questions with information and communication.

Varying kinds of management styles and skills came into play as the sites were developed, and these styles and skills tended to be more or less appropriate at different stages of the organization's development. Program sponsors frequently hired or assigned responsibilities for practice development to people whose skills were believed to be appropriate for the early stage of organizational development. This selection method did not necessarily ensure that an individual was capable of handling such managerial activities as developing the center's records and management information systems, projecting and monitoring the budget or generally implementing the program objectives. In some cases, the manager was a provider (a physician or physician extender) who was selected on the basis of clinical skills and then expected to exhibit some fairly technical managerial skills that changed over time.

The IAPC practice organizations experienced different organizational needs at different points in their development. This experience suggests that sponsors and managers must be sensitive, flexible and professional when addressing the changing requirements of the administrator role description. They also must recognize that the level of sophistication required to manage within the sponsoring organization's mature management structure differs from the level required at a primary care practice organization. These differences made it difficult in the IAPC experience for one individual to fluctuate between two settings and effectively manage two sets of priorities.

Another management issue observed at IAPC sites was the different styles and skills used by administrators when working with a community board. In many cases, the administrator helped the board conceptualize the various organizational stages of the practice and identify board functions and activities appropriate for these stages. This became an exercise in communication and feedback at different points in time as the board/administrator fit was determined. A few IAPC administrators worked with their boards to formally evaluate both this fit and their own administrative performance, which proved to be an effective process for IAPC practice growth.

A final consideration in practice management was the administrator's relationship with the practice physician(s). Based on IAPC experience, site physicians frequently were unaware of or did not appreciate the administrator's role. The administrators, because of their lack of experience with physicians, often found it difficult to assert themselves with the physicians in establishing and explaining administrative systems and monitoring center performance.

Physician Role

The advent of primary care organizations in the 1970s added two new facets to the physician's role: employee and manager. In the majority of rural primary care practices established in the 1970s, physicians were salaried employees in a practice owned and operated by nonphysicians, such as community boards, hospitals and other institutions. In others, physicians owned and operated the practice organization, which meant they were providers as well as employers. Most of the physicians who entered into these organizational roles had little training or experience with them or with the relationships they entailed, such as with community boards, hospital and medical practice administrators, federal agencies and private foundations. In general, the physicians at the IAPC sites were no exception.

For the most part, IAPC physicians were young and recent graduates of residency training programs. They typically were hired into the practice with little, if any, opportunity to participate in planning or goal-setting activities. Many physicians showed little interest and initiative in office management or team development and generally were not encouraged to do so by members of the organization. The physicians rarely related such issues as management by objectives, accountability, productivity, self-sufficiency or team building to the practice of medicine.

The IAPC experience does suggest, however, that as rural practices mature and as physicians and administrators gain more confidence and experience in this area, physician participation in organizational issues will expand as their roles and future within the primary care practice setting take shape. This is likely true both for physicians in private practice, which is clearly the dominant mode of physician organization in this country, and for physicians employed in a primary care organization. The practice of medicine is becoming increasingly regulated, competitive and accountable to a variety of organizations and clients. These conditions require skills in organizational behavior if effective coalitions with communities and consumers are to be built on both a group and an individual basis (Kaiser, 1981).

Finally, IAPC physicians increasingly perceived themselves as educators as well as providers. Doing so tended to enhance their capacity for professional leadership and their willingness to assume responsibilities in helping to determine organizational goals and objectives. It is likely that some of the physicians began to recognize that the investment of responsibility in shaping the practice organization translates into an investment in the physician's own future while creating a stronger incentive for retaining other providers within the practice organization.

Financing

The Innovations in Ambulatory Primary Care project grants totaled approximately $150,000 per site over the three-year period. The grant amount was purposely kept at a reasonable level in order to facilitate replication of the program in other rural communities with limited resources. The grants were intended to be joint ventures—the local community and the sponsoring organization pooling their respective resources and using the grant money to implement their plan. In addition to foundation funds, all IAPC sites obtained small amounts of in-kind (that is, service) or financial resources from their communities and/or sponsoring organizations. The financial contributions typically were used for facility acquisition and/or renovation. Five of the IAPC sites received major federal demonstration dollars in addition.

One of the earliest major concerns in IAPC site start-up was the facility in which to house the practice. The IAPC grants did not provide capital dollars for construction, renovation or major equipment. At most IAPC sites, responsibility for the facility was shared by the community and the sponsor. Seven communities raised funds and secured a mortgage for a new facility, using temporary quarters in the interim; seven other communities renovated an existing building for the facility.

Once the facility issue was resolved, financing concerns focused on operations and reimbursement. Institutional sponsors (hospital and university sponsors) fared better than community corporation sponsors did in terms of recovering practice site expenses through charges. At the end of the first year of grant funding, institutional-sponsored sites recovered an aggregate of 54 percent of expenses through charges; the community-sponsored sites recovered 43 percent. By the end of the second year, institutional sponsors had greatly improved that position, recovering 74 percent of expenses compared with the community sponsors' 48 percent. By the end of the third year of IAPC funding, those institutional sponsors receiving third-year funding recovered 85 percent of expenses compared with the community sponsors' 61 percent. On the other hand, success of the collection effort did not vary as greatly with sponsorship. The collection rate for institutional sponsors averaged 83 percent in both year 1 and year 2, while community sponsors collected 72 percent of charges in year 1 and 79 percent during year 2.

After three years of start-up, several sites achieved what they considered to be practice viability through a change from a nonprofit organizational status to a for-profit private group practice arrangement. Others considered the practice a viable entity when they achieved operational recognition within the county health department's approved budget. Still others bridged the gap between patient revenues and practice expenses by obtaining educational subsidies from the sponsoring organization in exchange for training site experience for medical students and residents.

The IAPC practice sites demonstrated that new medical practices and medical practice organizations can be initiated with a relatively small financial subsidy in areas where traditional medical care is declining and that the majority of these organizations will increase their productivity and financial stability over time. In general, long-range viability requires that sites not only increase their patient loads to service capacity but also increase their market shares. An improved self-sufficiency ratio (collected revenues to expenses) and a planned margin for growth will be crucial to the long-range viability of the IAPC sites.

Community Responsiveness

Rural primary care practices market "service delivery"; that is, services plus the attributes of the practice environment and the service delivery. Service delivery involves several factors: scope of services available onsite and through organizational linkages; staff professionalism—from the provider's credentials through the billing process; the nature and warmth of staff as well as of the facility; continuity and stability of both services and provider/patient relationships; patient familiarity with the surroundings and the process of patient treatment; and convenience of practice location and hours of business. It is possible that, by developing any of these service delivery factors, a new practice organization can gain an edge over existing patterns.

Marketing activities by IAPC sites typically constituted an individual consumer pursuit; that is, experiences were related by word of mouth from person to person. Consequently, every person associated with the organization and connected to the practice became a marketing tool in the community. One marketing technique used most successfully was to involve and thoroughly inform a community group and then use that group as marketing agents in the larger community. The group in turn provided feedback to IAPC practice personnel regarding community impressions and needs.

This marketing technique was particularly important for IAPC practice sites that had a community image of serving a particular population segment within that community (for instance, the indigent or the migrant population). However, because patient population bases were too small for most IAPC sites to maintain high quality and comprehensive services for select portions of the population and still achieve financial viability, it was important to market services to the entire community, including self-pay and insured segments.

Local community/consumer groups at IAPC sites were not seeking power or control when they organized, but rather seemed anxious to be able to voice their concerns about the diminishing or unsatisfactory health care conditions in their community and/or about recruiting a physician. Community control through formal nonprofit incorporation was viewed by the communities as a positive step in gaining access to the system and to additional health care resources.

The first hurdle for IAPC community board members was the conceptual shift from volunteer to "trustee"/director; from concerned citizen to responsible agent; from fund raising to policy formation. The next hurdle was the shift from individual to group process. Group decision making, risk-taking and financial understanding taxed even the most committed and concerted board and administrative efforts during the start-up period.

Despite the frustration of years of trial and error and unsettling change, the IAPC community governing boards contributed to the evolution of a meaningful and increasingly broader consumer role in the health care system. It is perhaps noteworthy that only one of the IAPC community-sponsored sites evolved into a physician-owned practice through a decision by the community board. These and other experiences will add to current knowledge about consumer involvement in health care delivery. In fact, a secondary effect of the rural primary care practice development efforts during the 1970s was to increase consumer awareness of and confidence in their ability to deal with the health care system.

Conclusions

Although these findings have been discussed in tentative terms, the perspective to be gained from the IAPC project is that the sites have been successful in many respects. A great deal of primary medical care is being delivered in rural areas where there was little or none before. Large and small organizations have been responsive to the medical care needs of small rural communities. And rural communities, leaders and provider institutions have learned a great deal and have undergone significant growth in the process.

The findings presented here, combined with other experiences from the rural health care initiatives of the 1970s, indicate the following conclusions about rural primary care delivery:

☐ Increasing the number of physicians in itself does not alleviate rural human resource shortages or access to care problems. However, there has been progress toward increasing the number of physicians choosing primary care and a rural location for practice and toward enhancing the opportunities for mid-level practitioners in rural areas.

☐ The development of organized practice settings has been a

relatively successful innovation in rural communities, both in enhancing physician recruitment and in gaining a cross-section of community support.

☐ Developmental funding was crucial in bringing hundreds of rural primary care practice opportunities into the mainstream of the health care delivery system. Examining the reimbursement system could be the key to long-term viability of these new practices. In the meantime, financial resource planning is a critical managerial task in striving for practice viability.

☐ Community involvement has proven to be an important marketing approach for rural primary care practices. Community boards of directors significantly advanced consumer education. In many cases, community initiative was the primary impetus in the development of the practice organization.

☐ The long-range viability of rural primary care practice organizations is ultimately connected with the capacity of their directors and/or managers to conceptualize the strategic framework within which the practice organization evolved and exists and to plan for and manage the organization from a long-range perspective. This planning need not be complex or conceptually overwhelming. It should, however, involve more than any one individual's goals and assessment of the environment.

The vast majority of business in the health care system is small business, and despite the trend toward multi-institutional systems, much health care delivery will remain small business. Yet relatively little is described in the literature about the issues or problems of small business enterprises and their position in the future. The experiences of the small, rural primary care practice sites that have evolved in a relatively short period of time provide valuable lessons to be learned.

References

Berney, B. The rise and fall of the UMW Fund. *South. Exposure*, 6(1978):95.

Clarke, L.J., and others. The impact of Hill-Burton: An analysis of hospital bed and physician distribution in the United States, 1950-1970. *Med. Care*, 18(1980):532.

Coleman, S. *Physician Distribution and Rural Access to Medical Services*. Santa Monica, CA: The Rand Corporation, 1976.

Copp, J.H. Diversity of rural society and health needs. In E.W. Hassinger and L.R.

Whiting (eds.), *Rural Health Services: Organization, Delivery and Use.* Ames, Iowa: Iowa State University Press, 1976.

Corwin, E.H.L. *The American Hospital.* New York: The Commonwealth Fund, 1946.

Falk, I.S. Financing for the reorganization of medical care services and their delivery. *Milbank Mem. Fund Q.,* 50(1972):191.

Geyman, J.P. Changing national priorities in medical education and primary care. *J. Fam. Pract.,* 8(1979):1117.

———. Family practice in evolution: Progress, problems, and projections. *N. Engl. J. Med.,* 298(1978):593.

Goldsmith, S.B. *Ambulatory Care.* Germantown, MD: Aspen Systems, 1977.

Jonas, S., and Rimer, B. Ambulatory Care. In S. Jonas (ed.), *Health Care Delivery in the U.S.* New York: Springer Publishing Co., 1977.

Kaiser, L.R. The physician in group practice: The personal challenge. *Group Pract. J.,* 30(1981):7.

Kane, R., and others. An evaluation of rural health care research. *Eval. Q.,* 3(1979):139.

———. Mail-order medicine: An analysis of the Sears Roebuck Foundation's Community Medical Assistance Program. *J. Am. Med. Assn.,* 232(1975):1023.

———. *An Overview of Rural Health Care Research.* Santa Monica, CA: The Rand Corporation, 1978.

Lane, S. Financing rural health services. In E.W. Hassinger and L.R. Whiting (eds.), *Rural Health Services: Organization, Delivery, and Use.* Ames, Iowa: Iowa State University Press, 1976.

Lewis, C.E., and others. *A Right to Health: The Problem of Access to Primary Medical Care.* New York: John Wiley & Sons, 1976.

Lichty, S.S., and Zuvekas, A. Rural health: Policies, progress and challenges. *Urban Health,* 9(1980):26.

Madison, D.L., and Bernstein, J.D. Rural health care and the rural hospital. In J. Bryant and others (eds.), *Community Hospitals and Primary Care.* Cambridge, MA: Ballinger Publishing Co., 1976.

McNerney, W.J., and Reidel, D.C. *Regionalization and Rural Health Care.* Ann Arbor: The University of Michigan, 1962.

Mott, F.D., and Roemer, M.I. *Rural Health and Medical Care.* New York: McGraw-Hill, 1948.

Parker, A.W. The dimensions of primary care: Blueprints for change. In S. Andreoipoulos (ed.), *Primary Care: Where Medicine Fails.* New York: John Wiley & Sons, 1974.

Penchansky, R., and Thomas, J.W. The concept of access: Definition and relationship to consumer satisfaction. *Med. Care,* 19(1981):127.

Ricketts, T.C., and others. Some unintended consequences of health insurance: The case of rural-urban subsidization. Unpublished paper, Health Services Research Center, University of North Carolina at Chapel Hill, June 1979.

Roemer, M.I. *Rural Health Care.* St. Louis: C.V. Mosby Co., 1976.

Rosenblatt, R.A., and Moscovice, I. The growth and evolution of rural primary care practice: The National Health Service Corps experience in the Northwest. *Med. Care,* 16(1978):819.

—————. The National Health Service Corps: Rapid growth and uncertain future. *Milbank Mem. Fund Q.,* 58(1980):283.

Rushing, W.A., and Wade, G.T. Community-structure constraints on distribution of physicians. *Health Serv. Res.,* 8(1973):283.

Schonfeld, W., and others. Organizational form in rural primary care: A typology. Paper presented at American Public Health Association annual meeting, 1981.

Sheps, C.G., and Bachar, M. Rural areas and personal health services: Current strategies. *Am. J. Public Health,* 71(1978):71.

Stevens, R. *American Medicine and the Public Interest.* New Haven: Yale University Press, 1971.

Woolf, M.A., and others. Demographic factors associated with physician staffing in rural areas: The experience of the National Health Service Corps. *Med. Care,* 19(1981):444.

2
Organizational Design and the Management of Primary Care Services

Arnold D. Kaluzny, Ph.D.
Thomas R. Konrad, Ph.D.

Dr. Kaluzny is a professor in the Department of Health Policy and Administration, School of Public Health, at the University of North Carolina, Chapel Hill.

Dr. Konrad is a research associate for the Health Services Research Center at the University of North Carolina.

Organizational Design and the Management of Primary Care Services

Rural primary care programs often are developed in social as well as geographic isolation. In attempting to develop programs and resolve problems, committed individuals sometimes are unaware of the challenges confronting similar programs in other communities and the efforts expended to meet those challenges. One consequence of this isolation is that program managers typically focus on individuals and personalities rather than on systematic organizational issues when confronting the everyday challenges and the periodic crises that occur in primary care programs. Although charisma and creativity are factors in behavioral explanations, defining programs solely in terms of personal characteristics limits a manager's understanding of a situation as well as his or her ability to intervene in an effective way.

Current thinking (Katz and Kahn, 1980) suggests that organizational characteristics are critical predictors of productivity, efficiency, innovation and survival. Health services research, for example, indicates that differences among physicians do not account for as much variance in selected performance indicators as do the characteristics of the organizational structure within which they function (for example, Rhee, 1977, 1976; Flood and Scott, 1978). Palmer and Reilley (1979) cite the importance of organizational characteristics as applied to quality assurance activities:

> Changing the process of care at the individual level is not the only nor necessarily the best way of improving quality of care. To the extent that structural characteristics (design characteristics) determine the quality of care, efforts to improve care in the long run through changing the structure of care (design) may prove to be more cost-effective than short run quality assurance programs. [p. 714]

This chapter examines organizational design as one set of organizational characteristics affecting the provision of primary care services. Specifically, the chapter: defines the basic elements and relationships involved in organizational/program design and discusses their implications for the provision of primary care services; uses these design elements and relationships to describe four basic types of primary care programs, identifies environmental factors affecting their development and operations and assesses the resulting managerial issues and roles associated with each type of program; and identifies major managerial approaches used in designing primary care programs and the implications of each approach for resolving important managerial issues.

What Is Organizational Design?

Organizational design is the arrangement of and the process of arranging structural characteristics to improve the efficiency, effectiveness, adaptability and survival of the organization (Kilmann, 1977). These arrangements involve a complex set of activities, roles, positions, information, people, equipment, work groups and subsystems. In a sense, these arrangements represent the basic anatomy and physiology of the organization.

Understanding the anatomy and physiology of an organization begins with the concept of viewing an organization (in this case a primary care program) as an open system. *Figure 1* indicates that the program has three major components: environment, design and performance.

Performance obviously results from program activities and constitutes that component to which all other components relate. However, performance and design must be understood within the context of

Figure 1 Organizational Components of a Primary Care Program

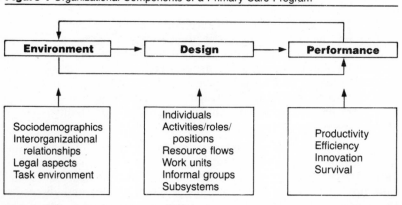

program environment. Environment is distinguished at several levels, including the larger economic, political and cultural context; the configuration of the organization and personal contacts affecting the program; and the immediate task environment, composed of resources that directly influence the program's ability to provide primary care services.

Although each of these three program components is worthy of detailed examination, the purpose of this chapter is to assess the organizational design component of primary care programs. While the concept of organizational design is more apparent in large-scale complex organizations, it is equally important when attempting to understand small-scale organizations with limited resources, such as primary care programs. In both large and small organizations, design provides the mechanism by which individuals are linked in collective activity to perform some socially valued activity—in this case the provision of primary care services. These services are not provided through a set of arrangements by which people act in a parallel manner; rather, they are provided through sets of people linked to each other and to the larger environment in complex ways, thereby directly affecting the kind, quantity and quality of the services provided. *Figure 2* presents a model of the major program design elements relevant to this discussion.

The key features in Figure 2 are the resource flows of interlocking people, funds, patients, equipment and information. These flows

Figure 2 Elements of Organizational Design

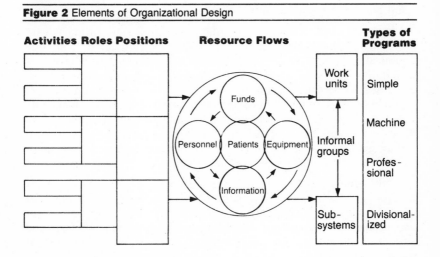

represent an ongoing set of transactions to which all roles, positions and activities relate and from which emerge work groups and subsystems unique to the particular program. Four organizational types, corresponding to the basic types of primary care programs, can be derived from the variations that occur when these work groups and subsystems interact. These organizational types are: community-sponsored; public sector-sponsored; provider-sponsored; and hospital-sponsored.

Basic Design Elements and Relationships

Roles refer to a set of activities or expected behaviors of an individual within the organization (Katz and Kahn, 1978). Roles are the building blocks of organizations, linking an individual's activities to the activities of others in the organization.

At the simplest level, an individual is expected to perform and actually does perform a set of related activities. For example, a nurse in a primary care program is expected to routinely distribute medications, order certain procedures and monitor the patient care process. Individuals, however, often perform several roles. For example, the receptionist may be responsible for scheduling patient referral appointments at a distant medical center, operating an x-ray machine and providing patient transportation in addition to performing routine clerical tasks. As the number of roles increases, the probability becomes greater that the individual will experience role conflict. This is further complicated by the fact that work roles constitute only a small part of the total number of roles played by an individual.

A specialized role of particular importance to primary care programs is the boundary role in which an individual from one organization interacts with constituents in that organization as well as with individuals from other organizations with a similar set of constituents (Adams, 1976). Because most primary care programs are relatively small, many individuals in these organizations occupy boundary role positions. For example, program managers interact with individuals in their own program as well as with their counterparts in various health service agencies. Similarly, many nurses interact with their colleagues as well as with counterparts in other organizations.

Individuals performing in boundary role positions experience different expectations and problems than do individuals not involved in such activities. They are responsible for representing, if not presenting, the "image" of their program to outsiders. Through the boundary role person, outsiders form their views and expectations of the program.

In addition, individuals in boundary role positions often are more closely involved in the program's environment than in the program itself. As a result, their orientation and identity may differ from those of other program personnel, generating suspicion among colleagues about their loyalty. Finally, persons in boundary role positions also can expect to encounter a great deal of conflict and ambiguity as part of their activities, a situation further complicated by the contradictory expectations of various constituencies. On the other hand, boundary roles can be used creatively to facilitate interorganizational communication and solidarity.

Positions refer to clusters of roles intended for one individual that locate the individual in organizational space. In the simplest case, a set of activities defines one role in one position; for example, the position of a staff nurse in a primary care program may entail only clinical activities and therefore represents one role in one position. Nurse involvement with clinical as well as managerial activities illustrates multiple roles in a single position.

Activities and *resource flows* refer to the specific tasks conducted within any given role that affect personnel, patients, funds, equipment and information. The patterning of these elements results in the development of work units and subsystems. For example, a specific work unit would be composed of a group of nurses who regularly perform general physical examinations of children, exchange information about their patients, use equipment and are paid for these activities. Several work units performing similar tasks involving an exchange of resource flows constitute a subsystem.

Work units refer to the organizational clustering of positions within the program. These may be characterized by:

☐ *Vertical differentiation,* which refers to the number of hierarchical levels or the "stacking" of organizational positions in the program. The higher the stack, the greater the degree of vertical differentiation. Using this concept, programs are often characterized as being "flat" or "tall," depending upon the height of the stack. (See *Figures 4a* and *5a* for examples of a tall and a flat program.)

☐ *Horizontal differentiation,* which refers to the clustering of positions into groupings or departments. Clustering may be based on purpose, function, place, time or type of clientele.

☐ *Integration,* which refers to the degree of collaboration among the program's differentiated positions and work units. The greater the differentiation among units, the greater the need for integration. Integration may be achieved through a number of mechanisms, including specifically designed units or teams to coordinate roles as well as managerial plans and procedures in differentiated departments (Lorsch, 1976; Lawrence and Lorsch, 1967).

☐ *Stratification,* which refers to the social distance separating positions within the program. The degree of social distance may vary greatly depending on the program or the particular functional grouping within the program. For example, the hospital administrator in a hospital-sponsored program is widely separated from the nurse practitioner at the health center. As a result, their orientations toward various program aspects may differ.

In addition to formal work units, programs may have a mosaic of interlocking informal groups. Although somewhat elusive, these groups are composed of individuals who derive mutual satisfaction from an interaction that is independent of the group's contribution to ongoing program activities. An informal group might consist of people who frequently eat lunch together and discuss organizational issues. Because this satisfaction from interaction may be of a purely personal nature or may in fact provide the basis for accomplishing specific objectives, the group may either facilitate or impede program operations.

Subsystems refer to the clustering of those activities that affect program resource flows and the interrelationships among work units (Katz and Kahn, 1978). They include*:

☐ *Production subsystem,* which refers to those work group activities that comprise the major program functions. In the case of primary care programs, the production subsystem involves those recurring activities concerned with the direct provision of patient care.

☐ *Maintenance subsystem,* which refers to those work group activities concerned with ensuring operational predictability and stability. For example, the development of a personnel department represents a cluster of activities to ensure the recruitment, training and maintenance of program personnel for the organization.

☐ *Adaptive subsystem,* which refers to those work group activities concerned with ensuring program adaptation to the changing demands and expectations of the community. For example, the

---

*A fifth subsystem, the supportive subsystem, has been eliminated to simplify this discussion.

operation of a planning committee within a primary care program represents an attempt to systematically evaluate changes in disease patterns or in public expectations about health services. Unfortunately, most primary care programs have not developed adaptive subsystems to evaluate environmental changes or systematic programs and technologies to accommodate these changes.

☐ *Managerial subsystem,* which refers to those work group activities concerned with coordinating and controlling the activities of the other subsystems. Ideally, the managerial subsystem cuts across all other subsystems and provides the basic integrity for the program as a whole. However, the particular stage of program development and the way in which various program subsystems are linked will often affect the ability of the managerial subsystem to function within the organization.

Subsystem Development

While four subsystems have been identified, their actual presence and operation will vary among primary care programs. These subsystems can be readily identified in some programs, while in others the subsystems may be embryonic or nonexistent. Because the same people often function in several different subsystems, the boundaries between subsystems can be hazy in small-scale organizations such as primary care programs.

Programs begin with the recognition that existing primary care services are inadequate or inaccessible and the initiation of a set of cooperative activities to provide improved services. This cooperative activity represents a primitive production subsystem (stage 1) of the type found in many rural community-sponsored primary care programs (Katz and Kahn, 1978).

A production subsystem must continually increase its level of performance reliability as it functions over time. This results in the development of managerial and maintenance subsystems (stage 2). The managerial subsystem provides a mechanism for formulating and enforcing rules to ensure that activities are performed in a predictable manner. Activities once representing simple responses to environmental demands subsequently represent a predetermined set of operations to accomplish some objective.

To ensure continued predictability, it is important that individuals are recruited and socialized into the program and that rewards and sanctions are administered in a predictable fashion. This predictability is accomplished through a set of specialized personnel activities and illustrates the maintenance subsystem (stage 3).

The final stage stems from the program's need to adapt to changes in the environment. Shifts in populations, changes in disease patterns and variations in funding sources illustrate important environmental factors that must be continually monitored and accommodated if the primary care program is to function effectively over time. This monitoring is accomplished through the development of adaptive subsystems (stage 4) such as long-range planning committees, community advisory boards or regular sources of technical assistance. Programs failing to develop adaptive subsystems may discover that the demand or need for their services no longer exists.

The sequential development of various subsystems has important implications for understanding the operation and problems of primary care programs. First, primary care programs often exist and operate at different stages in the development sequence. Failure to recognize the stage of development can result in unrealistic expectations both within the organization and on the part of the constituents with which the organization interacts. For example, while many primary care programs are at stage 1 in the developmental sequence, external funding agencies may assume that they are operating at stage 2 or 3—that is, with a fully developed managerial subsystem. This is illustrated by the problem encountered by many small programs when attempting to conform to the Bureau's Common Reporting Requirements (BCRR) developed by the federal Bureau of Community Health Services (Siegal, 1979). The BCRR, an accounting system developed primarily from experiences of urban community health centers, is viewed by many rural clinics as irrelevant given the realities of their situation and as being even less useful as a tool for internal monitoring or control (in other words, as a maintenance subsystem).

Second, primary care programs often fail to develop an adaptive subsystem. For example, many primary care programs serve specific population groups (such as migrant workers), and any change in the population will erode the patient base and threaten the survival of the program. While new or other markets may be available, the program lacking an adaptive subsystem will be unaware of their existence and therefore unable to redirect its activities.

Subsystem Linkages

Relationships among subsystems are as problematic as their development. Even when primary care programs operate with a fully developed set of subsystems, these subsystems may not always be tightly related to each other or represent an integrated whole. As Weick (1976) points out, many organizations are "loosely coupled"; that is, the various subsystems are tenuously related and, although "somehow attached," each subsystem retains some identity and separateness. The attachment may be circumscribed, infrequent, weak in mutual effects, unimportant or slow in response.

In primary care programs, loosely coupled relationships exist most commonly between the production and managerial subsystems. Production activities associated with patient care are based on specific technology that requires the extensive training and specialized skills of physicians and other primary care providers. This kind of production subsystem tends to be both self-limited and self-controlled and is organized around its own technical requirements and activities. The managerial subsystem, even when fully developed, may have only a tangential relationship with production activities, thus limiting its overall impact. This is common in primary care programs staffed by one or more National Health Service Corps (NHSC) providers. In such a situation, the managerial subsystem may be able to guide or coordinate day-to-day activities, but will encounter serious difficulty in developing or enforcing productivity norms or job descriptions since management has virtually no influence over the career contingencies of its assigned (NHSC) staff. The consequences of a "loosely coupled" managerial and production subsystem are illustrated in the Hemmingford case study.

Organizational Design Types Applied to Primary Care Programs

The existence of work units and subsystems and the manner in which they interact provide the basis for understanding the various types of primary care programs.* Figures 3 through 6 illustrate the relationships among the various design elements and characterize four basic types of primary care programs: (1) community-sponsored; (2) public sector-sponsored; (3) provider-sponsored; and (4) hospital-

---

*A similar but expanded typology applicable to all organizations is presented by Mintzberg (1979). Previous typologies characterizing primary care programs have used the underlying dimension of scale or size (Davis and Marshall, 1977; Yanni, 1978; Arthur Young and Associates, 1973). Characterizations of primary care programs in terms of sponsorship have been done by Durmaskin and others, 1979; Abt Associates, 1980; and Sheps and Bachar, 1981.

sponsored. Each type of program is described in terms of its design characteristics, environmental factors and those management issues associated with institutionalization, control, conflict and innovation.

These management issues represent the dominant problems that confront a primary care program manager as the program develops and functions. *Institutionalization* is that process by which a primary care program becomes an integral and accepted part of the community. *Control* is the process of intentionally influencing the behavior of persons, groups or organizations (Tannenbaum, 1969). *Innovation* is the process of adopting ideas or techniques or rearranging existing program elements in a fashion that is new to the existing structure (Zaltman and others, 1972). *Conflict* refers to various kinds of opposition and antagonistic interaction of the program with its environment, as between groups or subsystems within the program (Robbins, 1974).

Simple Structure: Community-Sponsored Primary Care Programs

Many primary care programs are best described as simple structures. These organizations consist of people engaged in cooperative activities to meet the community's need for primary care services. As *Figure 3a* shows, positions within the simple structure are characterized by limited vertical and horizontal differentiation; that is, there are few hierarchical levels and few departments or divisions. Positions are more likely to encompass multiple roles than would be the case in other types of primary care programs (for instance, in the Cape Meares case study, the nurse practitioner also is the program manager).

While degrees of stratification will depend upon the program, most community-sponsored primary care programs exhibit limited stratification. Integration is achieved through hierarchical relationships, but the entire structure is characterized by an overall commitment to providing primary care services. Because the program represents a cooperative activity, the community board plays an active role in program affairs at both the policy and administrative levels.

Figure 3b illustrates the simple structure in symbolic terms, highlighting the subsystems, resource flows and informal groups. Building on the basic organizational chart (Figure 3a) of the community-sponsored primary care program, the symbolic representation suggests that the program has a relatively primitive production subsystem (in other words, it has few services and/or few providers) and an emergent managerial subsystem that may or may not be loosely coupled to the production subsystem. Moreover, the resource flows

---

Figure 3a Simple Structure: Community-Sponsored Primary Care Program
(Conventional Model)

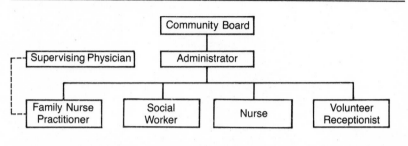

---

extend beyond the formal relationships between positions, giving rise to various informal groups throughout the organization. (These informal groups are separate from the formal relationships existing among positions.) It should be noted that, for purposes of clarity, the resource flows and informal groups shown in Figure 3b are merely illustrative; additional linkages would actually exist.

The major advantage of the simple structure is that it provides a mechanism for achieving a single objective. Individuals can readily identify with their tasks and achieve great satisfaction from their work since they perform critical roles in meeting program objectives.

The obvious disadvantage of the simple structure is that all production and managerial activities are performed by one or two individuals. As Mintzberg (1979) notes, "One heart attack can literally wipe out the organization's prime coordinating mechanism." Another disadvantage is the ease with which managerial personnel, particularly in a "tightly coupled" structure, can abuse that position. In this situation, subordinates lack appropriate alternatives or recourse and can only leave the organization if dissatisfied. Even the community board may be reluctant to terminate the manager or key provider since he or she may be the only person with adequate operating knowledge. The Cape Meares case study suggests such a dilemma.

Environmental Factors

Certain environmental characteristics will influence both a community's articulation of its need for primary health services as well as the range, sequence and timing of alternative organizational mechanisms used to provide those services. These characteristics include:

☐ Homogeneity of the community in terms of its socioeconomic, ethnic and residential stability factors;

Figure 3b Community-Sponsored Primary Care Program (Symbolic Model)

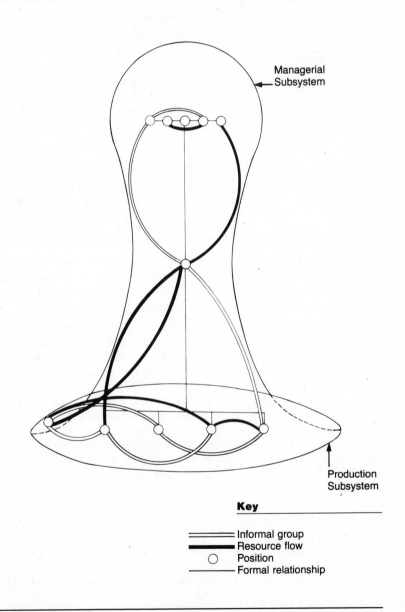

Managerial
Subsystem

Production
Subsystem

Key

═══ Informal group
━━━ Resource flow
○ Position
── Formal relationship

☐ Isolation of the community from larger population centers and health service organizations;

☐ Size of the community's population; and

☐ The community's previous experience with health service activities.

With few exceptions, community-sponsored primary care programs develop in an environment in which the community perceives a lack of health care services and pressures its leaders to respond. A history of scarce or intermittent availability of health care services in a small, isolated, homogeneous community can facilitate the creation of the local constituencies and coalitions necessary to support a primary care effort, as in the Hemmingford case study. Unfortunately, however, these same characteristics may hinder the development of the interorganizational relationships necessary for the long-term support of a primary care practice (such as, for referrals and hospital privileges).

Although a given community may be socially and economically homogeneous, both its health problems and the kinds of demands it makes upon the health care program can vary substantially. The task environment—emergency medical services, maternal and child health care services, substance abuse, care for the elderly—is probably as complex as that existing in a larger community. Yet the low volume of each type of clinical problem probably cannot justify differentiating the task structure into separate roles and positions; for example, by providing continuous services of an obstetrician, psychiatrist or ophthalmologist.

Two consequences flow from this situation. First, the program must possess a breadth of skills and array of interests capable of dealing with the full range of health problems. Second, the program must be able to develop linkages for referring patients to more specialized medical care and ancillary services. The development and particularly the formalization of these linkages require considerable managerial effort despite the apparent structural simplicity of the community-sponsored program.

Managerial Issues and Roles

The major issue confronting the simple structure of the community-sponsored primary care program is institutionalizing the program in the community. Institutionalization results from community acceptance and is usually measured in terms of the program's financial self-sufficiency.

Institutionalization is the primary responsibility of the program manager. Depending on when the manager joined the program, the diverse managerial role may involve everything from writing grant proposals to the more traditional managerial tasks of recruiting personnel, negotiating referral arrangements and mediating disagreements between the community board and the county medical society.

The manager's role in the community-sponsored program is complex and subtle. This is due, in part, to the fact that this role may be ill-defined or not sufficiently appreciated by the community board. The manager must be sensitive to local concerns—a sensitivity that often requires considerable time to develop, especially if the manager is a new community resident. Moreover, program goals and their relationship to the latent interests of board members must be thoroughly understood. Beneath the established organizational goals of primary care programs may exist broad social goals (such as the revival of the central business district) or even narrow personal motives (for example, the political ambitions of a board member or the maintenance of a local pharmacist's business). The manager must judge these latent goals critically to determine whether they enhance or undermine the program's stated objectives. Community boards must differentiate their broad policy-setting role from the manager's narrower administrative functions. In most cases, the manager must take the initiative in educating the board to this distinction and challenging them to act with this distinction in mind.

Board members also may have differing expectations—among themselves or with the manager—about the extent to which the program should achieve financial self-sufficiency and the time frame for achieving it. Consensus on these points is a prerequisite for effective management and long-range planning.

Machine Structure: Public Sector-Sponsored Primary Care Programs

Public sector programs are defined here as those programs sponsored by health departments. Many of these programs are best described as machine structures and are quite similar in structure to bureaucratic organizations. Positions are characterized by a high degree of vertical and horizontal differentiation and a high level of stratification. Integration occurs primarily through hierarchical relationships and formalized plans and procedures. *Figure 4a* illustrates the machine structure primary care program in conventional terms.

Figure 4b presents the public sector-sponsored program symbolically. Unlike the simple structure, the program has adaptive and

Figure 4a Machine Structure: Public Sector-Sponsored Primary Care Program (Conventional Model)

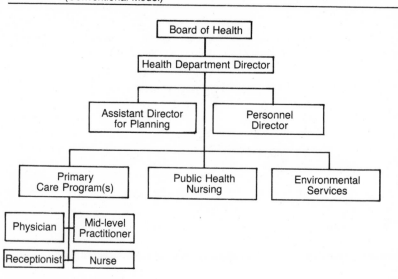

maintenance subsystems. All the subsystems are closely linked through resource flows, and the managerial subsystem dominates. Many informal groups operate thoughout the organization, transcending formal working relationships among positions. (Again, the resource flows and informal groups depicted are illustrative, since additional linkages would actually be present.)

The major advantage of the machine structure as a design for primary care programs is its ability to ensure accountability and predictability in use of resources. The development of all four subsystems and the dominance of the managerial subsystem with a tight coupling to the other three subsystems ensure a high level of control within the structure.

Accountability and predictability are not achieved without cost, however. The machine structure appears to operate without recognizing the unique contributions of individuals, who often are used as interchangeable parts within the system. Also, the quest for predictability often impedes the structure's ability to meet the varying needs of the clients or patients it was developed to serve. Human considerations often do not conform to the structural requirements for accountability and predictability. Although this problem often can be mitigated when program individuals go beyond their prescribed roles and

48

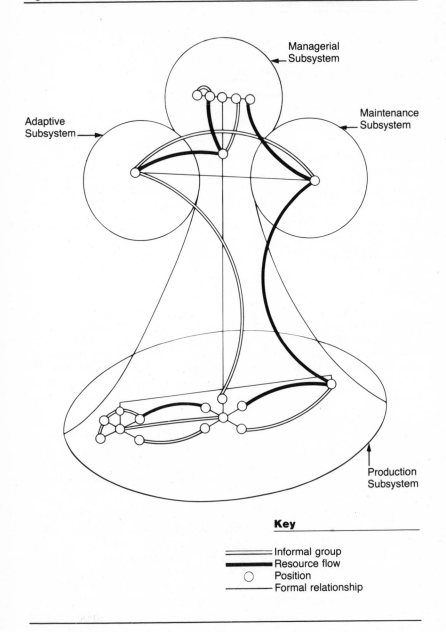

Figure 4b Public Sector-Sponsored Primary Care Program (Symbolic Model)

activities, it may require extra effort from already overwhelmed personnel. The informal groups that develop within this type of design do tend to provide a support structure that enables people to deal with unique problems as they arise. (An informal group might consist of people from different departments who frequently socialize together and discuss organizational issues.)

Environmental Factors

The pressure for work accountability and appropriate methods for ensuring this accountability are characteristic of public bureaucracies. Within the context of primary care programs, however, certain characteristics of the environment render these pressures and procedures particularly difficult to manage. First, the program's geographic service boundaries are likely to be mandated by the public health department's jurisdiction rather than by a logical market or service area for primary care.

Second, the task environment may be defined in such a way that primary care is treated as another categorical program at the "bottom" of the hierarchy (for example, see the Tehama County case study). The nature of traditional public health departments can easily subvert the comprehensiveness of primary care activities. To illustrate, one local health department director characterized his primary care program in the following way: "We don't treat patients here, we treat the plague." This inability to distinguish primary care from categorical programs makes primary care programs particularly vulnerable during periods of fiscal austerity.

Finally, although the public sector nature of the program may facilitate linkages with other health and social welfare workers and community programs, in doing so, the unique potential and contribution of primary care may be overlooked. Since the poor typically are the ones served by health department programs, the primary care program itself may be unable to overcome an image in the community as a "public clinic." Thus, while a patient base can be developed, a broader constituency that could perform effective advocacy or advisory functions for the program may be difficult to cultivate.

Managerial Issues and Roles

A major issue in the bureaucratically structured health department-sponsored program is control over the content of the primary care program. Although the health department's ability to absorb special program funds into routine operations can be exaggerated, there is no doubt that pressure exists to do just that. Hence, the managerial problems of developing and maintaining autonomy for primary care programs, as well as integrating existing categorical services into a primary care package, are paramount. The long tradition of health departments as complementary to, but not competitive with, private medical practice has made the provision of medical care a challenge for those health departments attempting to assume primary care responsibility for the general community.

The manager's role in a public sector-sponsored program is one of achieving and maintaining autonomy for the primary care program while ensuring that the program remains an integral part of the larger organization. In the Tehama County case study, where the primary care facility is located some distance from the health department's traditional base of operation while the program manager is located near the facility, an appropriate balance of autonomy and integration is easily achieved. However, where the primary care center is located in a health department facility, community and even staff recognition of the primary care function may be difficult to promote. Furthermore, role conflict may ensue if the manager is responsible for more than administering the primary care program.

Professional Structure: Provider-Sponsored Primary Care Programs

Provider-sponsored primary care programs illustrate the professional structure. As *Figure 5a* shows, positions within the structure are characterized by limited vertical differentiation and a high degree of horizontal differentiation; that is, the structure has relatively few layers despite the existence of many units within the organization, reflecting its complexity and overall level of specialization. Moreover, the dominance of medical professionals typically results in a high level of stratification among positions.

In the symbolic representation of this structure *(Figure 5b)*, the production subsystem is well-developed and loosely coupled to the managerial subsystem, while other subsystems are absent. The production subsystem dominates the structure, and although the managerial subsystem is present, it is often isolated from the organization's power base—that is, the physician group.

Despite these features, the professional structure provides a mechanism for dealing with complex activities. It provides the operating setting for physicians who have the special expertise to deal with complex patient care problems. This kind of structure, however, is often criticized as being unresponsive to patients and unaccountable to the community (Friedson, 1970). Because physicians are free to define

Figure 5a Professional Structure: Provider-Sponsored Primary Care Program (Conventional Model)

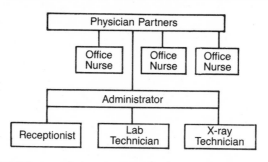

reality to fit their respective disciplines, problems can be overlooked or viewed as isolated acute episodes fitting only clinical categories.

Finally, where the professional structure fails to respond to patient and community needs, outsiders (clients, managers from machine structures and governmental representatives) may conclude that the structure is out of control and no longer accountable. This in turn leads external funding agencies to press for the adoption of managerial approaches more consistent with the machine structure; for example, direct supervision and the use of formal rules and regulations.

Environmental Factors

The most salient aspect of the environment for the provider-sponsored program is usually the preexisting medical community. An organized primary care center sponsored by a physician or physician group is generally more acceptable to the local medical community than are the other models. Although many factors may contribute to this acceptance, physician dominance of the organization is viewed as less threatening than other organizational arrangements. This acceptance also enables easier access to hospital facilities than do other organizational types.

The provider-sponsored program tends to relate to its community more as a "market area" than as a "service area." Specific geopolitical boundaries may define the service area of a public sector program, while the community-sponsored program usually has at least an implicit mandate to serve a geographically defined area. The provider-sponsored program, however, operates with greater flexibility in that it

Figure 5b Provider-Sponsored Primary Care Program (Symbolic Model)

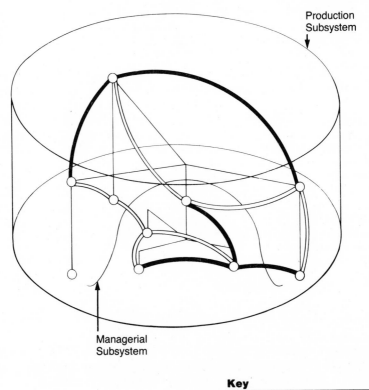

Production
Subsystem

Managerial
Subsystem

Key

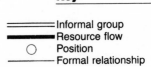

Informal group
Resource flow
○ Position
Formal relationship

can develop a clientele that may or may not be readily identifiable as a specific population. This flexibility enables the practice to adapt to rapidly changing community circumstances, including demographic shifts, changes in market patterns or travel networks. Such flexibility and autonomy may result in responsiveness to a market but not necessarily in accountability to or responsibility for a community.

Managerial Issues and Roles

Integration is extremely difficult to achieve in professional structures. Clinical professionals have little patience with or interest in direct program coordination since their interests lie in specific clinical tasks and the autonomy to complete those tasks.

Managers can provide integration by helping physicians negotiate within the larger health care system. For example, managers often can achieve credibility among physicians by negotiating programs or projects through "the system," thereby enhancing their ability to integrate and control the operations of the professional structure. As described by Mintzberg (1979, p. 211):

> . . . he (the professional) depends on the full-time administrator to help him negotiate his project through the system. For one thing, the administrator has time to worry about such matters—after all, administration is his job. . . . For another, the administrator has a full knowledge of the . . . system as well as many personal contacts within it, both of which are necessary to see projects through it. The administrator deals with the system every day; the professional entrepreneur may promote only one new project in his entire career. Finally, the administrator is more likely to have the requisite managerial skills, for example, those of negotiation and persuasion.

> But the power of the effective administrator to influence strategy goes beyond helping the professionals. Every good manager seeks to change his organization in his own way, to alter its strategies to make it more effective. In the Professional Bureaucracy, this translates into a set of strategic initiatives that the administrator himself wishes to take. But in these structures —in principle bottom up—the administrator cannot impose his will on the professionals of the operating core. Instead, he must rely on his informal power, and apply it subtly. Knowing that the professionals

want nothing more than to be left alone, the administrator moves carefully—in incremental steps, each one hardly discernible. In this way, he may achieve over time changes that the professionals would have rejected out of hand had they been proposed all at once.

A related managerial role in the provider-sponsored primary care program is developing and promoting innovative programs and expanding the traditional focus of the medical practice to include more comprehensive health service goals and objectives. However, the autonomous nature of physicians within the structure makes it difficult to achieve interdisciplinary programmatic innovations. Because each practitioner competes for resources, one may readily cancel out the others' efforts (Wilson, 1967). Innovation requires a good working relationship with the dominant providers and a commitment by the providers to support such activities. Conversely, the manager must be able to demonstrate how these innovations contribute to "practice building" for the physician and hence ensure long-term viability of the center as a medical practice entity. Although some evidence suggests that recently trained primary care physicians subscribe more readily to the ethos of comprehensive primary care, the manager must subtly engineer that commitment into concrete policies and plans.

Divisionalized Structure: Hospital-Sponsored Primary Care Programs

In this design, a larger corporate structure is superimposed on one or a number of small operating primary care programs to create a primary care system. *Figures 6a* and *6b* illustrate this design in both conventional and symbolic representations. These programs may take several different forms, as in the C.T. Meyer Hospital case study (a variation of the simple structure) and the University Medical Center case study (a divisionalized form of the professional structure).

Positions are characterized by a high degree of vertical and horizontal differentiation and a great deal of stratification. Integration is highly formalized and represented by specific departments or positions that coordinate activities at the corporate level as well as by role activities and formal procedures at the local program level. Because of the structure's greater overall scale and complexity, there can be great variability in the location of administrative responsibility for the primary care program and in the relationship between the primary care center and other activities of the larger organization. Such contrasting modes of integration in decentralized primary care

Figure 6a Divisionalized Structure: Hospital-Sponsored Primary Care Program (Conventional Model)

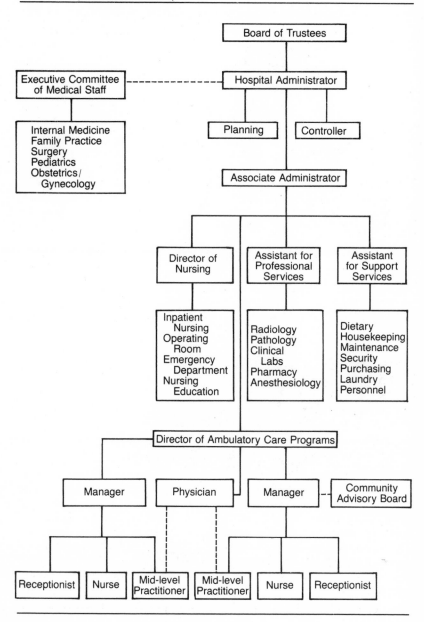

Figure 6b Hospital-Sponsored Primary Care Program (Symbolic Model)

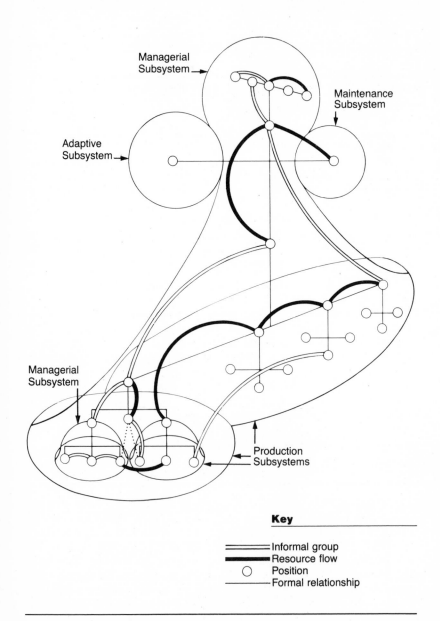

Managerial
Subsystem

Maintenance
Subsystem

Adaptive
Subsystem

Managerial
Subsystem

Production
Subsystems

Key

Informal group
Resource flow
○ Position
Formal relationship

programs are seen in the organizational structures of the University Medical Center, Montgomery County Hospital and Lakeview Hospital case studies.

Environmental Factors

The hospital-sponsored primary care program typically is located fairly close to other health care resources, since the primary care program's service area generally is defined as a portion of the sponsoring hospital's service area. The institutional rivalries of hospitals, well understood in urban areas, often are expressed as territorial rivalries in rural communities. Viewed from this perspective, the primary care center is a strategic outpost of the hospital and is designed to prevent patients from drifting off to another hospital's service area and to facilitate expansion into a new or shifting service area (for example, the Lakeview Hospital case study). Viewed from the primary care center's perspective, however, the sponsoring hospital dominates the environment, so that local concerns and program needs may be somewhat low on the sponsor's scale of priorities (as the University Medical Center and Montgomery County Hospital case studies suggest).

Hospital-sponsored programs that rely on physician residents from a primary care specialty training program to provide services face another environmental issue. Generally, program staffing is not problematic, and access to the hospital and a broad range of diagnostic and therapeutic capabilities is readily available. However, administrative coordination may be a problem because administrative responsibility for the residency program and for the primary care center is separated. In addition, community residents may be reluctant to use the program since they cannot identify with a specific provider to whom they can turn as "my doctor" and with whom they can experience a long-term relationship.

Managerial Issues and Roles

The hospital's ability to initiate and sponsor primary care programs carries both advantages and disadvantages. When the manager of the primary care program is part of the hospital's organizational hierarchy (for instance, an assistant administrator), that program has access to a number of resources frequently unavailable to a freestanding program. In the C.T. Meyer Hospital case study, for example, the program manager uses hospital data to define service areas and project utilization levels for satellite clinics. This benefit of a link to the sponsor organization is achieved at the price of an inherent conflict, however, between the goals of the hospital and the satellite primary care clinic. Although hospitals often are genuinely concerned with the adequate and effective provision of ambulatory care, most hospital administrators seek high occupancy rates. As a result, any satellite clinic oriented to preventive health care and the provision of ambulatory services in the local community in lieu of hospital referral for inpatient services will at some point come into conflict with the hospital itself. The manager occupying a boundary role between the primary care program and the hospital then becomes responsible for reconciling or controlling this conflict. The C.T. Meyer Hospital case study illustrates this kind of resource allocation conflict.

Because the divisionalized structure of the hospital-sponsored program is the most variable of the organizational designs, the manager's role in this setting will be the most complex and challenging since all the problems of institutionalization, control, innovation and conflict are likely to emerge. For example, in the Lakeview Hospital case study, the attempt to institutionalize the program in the original target community never succeeds. In the University Medical Center case study, the novelty of the organization's legal structure challenges the program's complex accountability structure, and the traditional university and hospital "adaptive subsystems" are slow in responding to the requirements of the primary care program. Finally, because this structure involves multiple parties (the hospital, its medical staff, the primary care staff, rotating residents, patients and community boards), negotiating requirements often tax the manager's skills and capabilities.

Managerial Design Perspectives

Primary care programs can be arranged or designed to contend effectively with problems of institutionalization, innovation, control and conflict. Simon (1969) notes that:

> Everyone designs who devises courses of action aimed at changing existing situations into preferred ones. The intellectual activity that produces material artifacts is no different fundamentally from the one that prescribes remedies for sick patients or the one that devises a new sales plan for a company or social welfare policy for a state. Design, so construed, is the core of all professional training; it is the principal mark that distinguishes the professionals from the scientists. Schools of engineering as well as schools of

> architecture, business, education, law and medicine
> are all centrally concerned with the process of design.
> [pp. 55-56]

Most primary care program managers pride themselves on their pragmatic orientation, but their design efforts occur within an uncertain environment, forcing them to adopt or develop—often through a process of trial and error—some theory or perspective to explain the internal workings of their organization. In essence, these are perspectives of the design process. Varying models, implicitly or explicitly derived, lead to different perceptions and conclusions (Elmore, 1978).

As Allison (1971) notes, "What we see and judge to be important depends not only on the evidence but also on the 'conceptual lens' through which we look at the evidence" [p. 2]. Several "conceptual lenses" or perspectives are currently available to guide the manager in designing primary care programs. The two discussed in this chapter are the rational and the ecological perspectives. Each provides a somewhat different explanation or highlights different primary care program design issues and emphasizes different factors important to resolving problems associated with institutionalization, control, innovation and conflict.

Rational Perspective

From the rational perspective, design is a conscious attempt to enhance some aspect of program activity with the underlying expectation that these changes will directly affect program performance. By and large, three approaches are dominant in this perspective: classical, behavioral and contingency. In each approach, the manager is viewed as a processor who responds to environmental demands and program constraints. From the rational perspective, the managerial function is to manipulate both resource flows and existing roles, activities and positions (and the resulting configurations) in ways that best meet program needs.

Classical Approach

The classical approach is perhaps the most widely accepted, at least implicitly, by managers of primary care programs. Under this approach, managers are responsible for defining policies, assigning responsibilities and ensuring staff performance accountability. Emphasis is on a set of management principles that, if followed, will enhance overall program performance. A few of the most commonly applied prescriptions are:

☐ An organization should have a hierarchy, sometimes referred to as "a scalar process," whereby lines of authority and responsibility extend upward and downward through several levels, with a broad functional base at the bottom and a single executive at the top.

☐ Without exception, every unit and person in the organization should be answerable ultimately to the chief executive officer, who occupies the supreme position in the hierarchy.

☐ The number of departments should be sufficiently small to permit an effective "span of control" for the chief executive officer, yet sufficiently large to provide effective contact with all major organizational functions.

Using these prescriptions, managers are able to explain the problems associated with various aspects of institutionalization, control, innovation and conflict as resulting from bad management practices. Bad management is defined as the manager's failure to clearly define the operational objectives of the program and apply appropriate management principles. For example, a control problem relates to the manager's failure to translate program goals into clear operational policies and, as a result, to hold individuals accountable for their actions. The solution is to increase the number of rules and regulations for program personnel.

The classical approach assumes a fixed quantity of control consistent with the formal hierarchy of the organization. Thus, supervisors and subordinates are engaged in a "zero-sum game" in which an increase in the level of control exercised by one party must be accompanied by a corresponding decrease in the level of control exercised by another party (Tannenbaum, 1969). It is beyond the scope of the classical approach to consider control as an indeterminate quantity pervading the organization, nor does it postulate that redistribution of control among parties may, in fact, enhance the overall level of control within the organization.

Public sector-sponsored programs tend to rely on the classical design perspective more often than do other primary care program models. Personnel accountability is the major strength of this approach. Its limitation, however, is an inability to effectively deal with the unforeseen and unanticipated human problems associated with primary care delivery. It also tends to overlook the role of informal groups in supporting or inhibiting the achievement of organizational goals.

The classical approach also offers a ready explanation for problems of innovation. Here the difficulty is typically attributed to "red tape" and the structure's failure to respond quickly to environmental demands. This is particularly true in less autonomous programs such as hospital-sponsored and public sector-sponsored. Managers using the classical approach attempt to resolve these problems and facilitate the innovation process by manipulating organizational guidelines, rules and regulations. These managerial interventions are likely to have little impact on physicians, however. Successful innovation requires recognition and ultimately acceptance by individuals who, over the years, have developed defense mechanisms to changes in guidelines, rules and regulations.

Behavioral Approach

The behavioral approach, in part a reaction to the development of classical management guidelines, views the problems facing a primary care program in a different way. Here, design focuses on fundamental assumptions about individuals within the organization. Individuals are considered capable of making appropriate choices and demonstrating growth and are thought to behave in response to both external stimuli and an inner thrust that makes each individual unique.

This approach provides a different view of the issue of control. Rather than emphasizing the manipulation of rules and regulations (thus enhancing the control aspects of the design), emphasis is on the expectations of individuals within the program. Individuals are expected to participate in various aspects of program decision making at all levels; and in order to avoid conflict, special attention is given to the nature of interpersonal relations.

Provider-sponsored programs tend to reinforce this approach to management. The physician's personality, professional inclinations and interests tend to dominate the manager's perception of what is occurring in the program. This approach easily leads to selective inattention to the structural aspects of the program. The manager may fail to recognize or express aspects of the program and the physician's career objectives that are mutually conflicting.

Contingency Approach

The logical outgrowth of the classical and behavioral orientations is the development of a contingency approach. Here, the design attempts to achieve a balance between community and program characteristics as well as between individual and program characteristics. When this balance occurs, there is an expected positive effect on the overall performance of the individual, the work unit and the organization.

When using a contingency approach in the design process, management would explain problems associated with innovation as a failure to appropriately identify the decision stage in the innovation process and to manipulate variables appropriate to that particular stage. For example, in the Montgomery County Hospital case study, funds to implement the primary care program are available before a consensus is reached on the long-term structure of the program. Similarly, problems associated with institutionalization would focus on basic problem characteristics vis-a-vis the environment in which the program currently operates. The different community development approaches used with the two satellite clinics in the C.T. Meyer Hospital case study illustrate this point. Enhancing institutionalization and making the program more compatible with its environment would require various modifications in basic structural characteristics.

A similar orientation is applied in dealing with issues of control and conflict. Unlike the behavioral approach, the contingency approach does not deny conflict but views it as a variable to be manipulated within the overall design of the program (Robbins, 1974). Similarly, control represents a method of matching individuals' characteristics with ongoing environmental or design characteristics (Lorsch, 1976). This perspective underlies the perpetual search for nurses and physicians with rural backgrounds to staff rural primary care centers.

Ecological Perspective

From the ecological perspective, program design is not the result of management's ability to manipulate roles, activities and positions, thereby enhancing program effectiveness, but instead is an outgrowth of the nature and distribution of environmental resources as well as the outcome of political contests within the program (Aldrich, 1979; Pfeffer and Salancik, 1978).

The manager's primary activity under this perspective is modifying the program's environment by manipulating those external constraints and resources that directly affect the program. The manager seeks to enact with or create an environment more favorable to the existing program design (Weick, 1969); moreover, managers give meaning to events in the environment only after they have occurred and make their decisions for the future on the basis of a selective perception of the total range of environmental events affecting the organization. This counters the more typical notion of managerial decision making as a forward-looking process. However, it should be remembered that future actions are always based on prior experience.

From this point of view, issues of institutionalization, control, innovation and conflict involve complex interaction with the program's environment. For example, problems of institutionalization are not confronted internally but by developing coalitions outside the organization that will support or enhance the program's operation. Similarly, some innovation and conflict issues can be resolved by acquiring more environmental resources, thereby facilitating the flow of activities and avoiding potentially competitive situations that arise when resources are scarce and diminishing.

Finally, the question of control also is addressed under this perspective by manipulating the external environment. Emphasis is placed on developing external groups that provide mutual support for primary care programs (such as state or national primary care associations or *ad hoc* lobbying groups to modify restrictive professional acts).

Conclusions

The design of primary care programs reflects basic trends in the larger health services system. Although this chapter has examined major design characteristics and resultant managerial issues associated with four major types of ongoing primary care programs, future trends in the design of these programs within the context of their evolutionary development also warrant consideration (Schonfeld and others, 1982).

Historically, community residents and health care policy makers defined primary care needs as a problem of maldistribution of health professionals, principally physicians. When defined in this manner, the solution was to increase the number of physicians whose background and training encouraged them to elect practice in rural areas and in primary care specialties. As a complementary solution, community efforts focused on "doctor search committees." But recent studies indicate that, while some redistribution of physicians has occurred, many communities still lack continuous primary care services.

Recognizing the limitations of this approach, policy makers shifted the initiative to developing sites that would attract and retain primary care providers. One example of this was the expanded role of the National Health Service Corps from personnel placement to a "staffing arm" of the Bureau of Community Health Services. During this period, various community and organizational development efforts resulted in the creation of many community-sponsored primary care programs. Although these were initiated with great expectations, problems have surrounded their attempts to achieve self-sufficiency and to develop and maintain linkages with institutional-based health care resources.

It now appears that future emphasis will be placed on the development of regional primary health care systems and on contract management arrangements for various types of primary care programs. These developments parallel the emergence of multihospital systems and the use of contract management services by hospitals.

The development of regional primary health care systems has taken two forms. The first is satellite facilities or extensions of previously existing health service delivery organizations. These may involve community hospital satellites (Madison and Bernstein, 1976), group practice satellites (Mikhaelevsky, 1973), health department satellite clinics and the large, comprehensive health center operating various service programs and several sites. The second involves a network of community-sponsored clinics. Generally, these networks are not initiated through the intervention or extension of larger medical care delivery organizations, but grow from a coalition of preexisting, autonomous, small-scale clinics (Sheps and Madison, 1977). They result from joint efforts by community leaders in several small proximate communities and the pooling of resources to develop organizational solutions to deficiencies in medical care services. Such efforts often are facilitated by third parties such as hospitals, health systems agencies or state primary care development agencies. However, the network typically is governed by a community board relatively independent of existing health care providers and institutions.

Managers of primary care programs must be aware of the historical basis of and future trends in the design of primary care services. These designs are dynamic, evolving over time and continually encountering problems and challenges associated with institutionalization, control, conflict and innovation. The particular sequence in which these issues are encountered, their dominance vis-a-vis other problems and how they are resolved depend on the type of program, its current stage of development and the particular design perspective held by relevant actors. As previously noted, issues of control and innovation dominate provider-sponsored and public sector-sponsored programs respectively; issues of institutionalization dominate community-sponsored programs; and issues of conflict are most prevalent in hospital-sponsored programs. Moreover, the particular design perspective used by managers and health care professionals may either facilitate or impede the recognition and/or resolution of these problems. For example, the ecological and contingency perspectives, with their emphasis on the environment and its relationship to program characteristics, appear to be more successful in achieving institutionalization than either the classical or behavioral perspective.

The small scale and apparent isolation of rural primary care programs can be deceptive. In reality, they are extremely complex, encompassing a variety of roles and activities in an ever-changing environment. An awareness of these relationships, coupled with an understanding of basic design elements and an explicit recognition of how particular design perspectives affect certain actions, will prevent managers and health service providers from inappropriately defining critical management issues in personality terms and disregarding important systematic properties of their programs. This recognition will help both managers and health care providers engaged in primary care to meet the challenges ahead.

References

Abt Associates. *A Study to Evaluate and Compare Four Organizational Approaches to the Delivery of Primary Health Care in the Appalachian Region.* Washington, DC: Appalachian Regional Commission, 1980.

Adams, S. The structure and dynamics of behavior of organizational boundary roles. In M. Dunnette (ed.), *Handbook of Industrial and Organizational Psychology.* Chicago: Rand McNally, 1976.

Aldrich, H. *Organizations and Environment.* Englewood Cliffs, NJ: Prentice-Hall, 1979.

Allison, G. *Essence of Decision: Explaining the Cuban Missile Crisis.* Boston: Little Brown, 1971.

Arthur Young and Associates. *Report on the Development of a Community-Health Care Delivery Matching Methodology.* National Health Service Corps Contract no. HSM 110—72—279, 1973.

Davis, K., and Marshall R. Health care for the medically underserved, Section 1502 (1). In *Papers on the National Health Guidelines: The Priorities of Section 1502.* (Publication no. [HRA] 77-641). Washington, DC: U.S. Dept. of Health, Education and Welfare, 1977.

Durmaskin, B., and others. *West Virginia Primary Care Clinics: Development, Availability, Utilization, and Service Area Determination for 1977 and 1978.* Morgantown, WV: Office of Health Services Research, West Virginia University, 1979.

Elmore, G. Organizational models of social program implementation. *Public Policy,* 26(1978):185.

Flood, A., and Scott, W.R. Professional power and professional effectiveness: The power of the surgical staff and quality of surgical care in hospitals. *J. Health Soc. Behav.*, 19(1978):240.

Friedson, E. *Professional Dominance: The Social Structure of Medical Care.* New York: Atherton, 1970.

Katz, D., and Kahn, R. Organizations as social systems. In E. Lawler and others (eds.), *Organizational Assessment: Perspectives on the Measurement of Organizational Behavior and the Quality of Work Life.* New York: Wiley-Interscience, 1980.

———. *The Social Psychology of Organizations.* New York: John Wiley & Sons, 1978.

Kilmann, R. *Social Systems Design.* New York: North-Hillard, 1977.

Lawrence, P., and Lorsch, J. *Organization and Environment: Managing Differentiation and Integration.* Boston: Harvard Business School, 1967.

Lorsch, J. Contingency theory and organizational design: A personal odyssey. In R. Kilmann and others (eds.), *The Management of Organizational Design.* New York: North-Hillard, 1976.

Madison, D., and Bernstein, J. Rural health care and the rural hospital. In J. Bryant and others (eds.), *Community Hospitals and Primary Care.* Cambridge, MA: Ballinger Publishing Co., 1976.

Mikhaelevsky, A. *Satellite Clinics.* Alexandria, VA: American Association of Medical Clinics, 1973.

Mintzberg, H. *The Structure of Organizations.* Englewood Cliffs, NJ: Prentice-Hall, 1979.

Palmer, R., and Reilley, M. Individual and institutional variables which may serve as indicators of the quality of medical care. *Med. Care,* 17(1979):693.

Pfeffer, J., and Salancik, G. *The External Control of Organizations.* New York: Harper and Row, 1978.

Rhee, S. Factors determining the quality of physician performance in patient care. *Med. Care,* 14(1976):733.

———. Relative importance of physicians' personal and situational characteristics for the quality of patient care. *J. Health Soc. Behav.,* 18(1977):10.

Robbins, A. *Managing Organizational Conflict.* Englewood Cliffs, NJ: Prentice-Hall, 1974.

Schonfeld, W., and others. A typology of practice organization in rural primary care. *Amer. J. Public Health* (in press).

Sheps, C., and Bachar, M. Rural areas and personal health services: Current strategies. *Amer. J. Public Health,* 71(1981):71.

Sheps, C., and Madison, D. The medical perspective. In E. Ginzberg (ed.), *Regionalization and Health Policy.* (Publication no. [HRA] 77-623). Washington, DC: U.S. Dept. of Health, Education and Welfare, 1977.

Siegal, J. *Report on the Results of a Survey of HURA and RHI Grant Recipients on the BCRR.* Waterville, ME: National Rural Primary Care Association, Dec. 7, 1979.

Simon, H. *The Sciences of the Artificial.* Boston: MIT Press, 1969.

Tannenbaum, A. *Control in Organizations*. New York: McGraw-Hill, 1969.

Weick, K. Educational organizations as loosely coupled systems. *Adm. Sci. Q.*, 21(1976):1.

————. *The Social Psychology of Organizing*. Reading, MA: Addison-Wesley, 1969.

Wilson, J. Innovation in organizations: Notes toward a theory. In J. Thompson (ed.), *Approaches to Organizational Design*. Pittsburgh: University of Pittsburgh Press, 1967.

Yanni, F. Primary care: Future directions or return to the basics. *Fam. Community Health*, 1(1978):27.

Zaltman, G., and others. *Innovation in Organizations*. New York: John Wiley & Sons, 1972.

3
Human Resource Planning and Management

Caryl E. Carpenter, M.P.H.

Ms. Carpenter is an instructor in the Health Services Management Section, School of Health Related Professions, at the University of Missouri, Columbia.

Human Resource Planning and Management

National attention recently has focused on the maldistribution of physicians and other health personnel. Many rural communities once served by general practitioners are now without ready access to medical care. This problem is related to increased medical specialization and a growing dependence by physicians on medical technology. Rural areas have experienced a loss of physicians as more physicians elect postgraduate specialty training. Because specialists require a larger population base for their practices, they tend to remain in urban and suburban areas upon completion of their training. Physicians trained in sophisticated teaching hospitals also become dependent on the resources of those institutions and tend to locate close to those resources.

The expectations of many rural areas have not changed in correspondence to these changes in medical education and practice. Rural health care consumers still seek the old health delivery prototype. Communities organize to build facilities and raise funds in the hope of attracting one or two physicians who will care for their families and always be available. Yet many communities still without physician coverage fail to recognize that their recruitment strategies are poorly designed and unrealistic given today's health care environment.

This chapter discusses the issues associated with recruiting and retaining health care professionals, especially physicians. A brief review of various public policy initiatives that were designed to remedy the health personnel distribution problem is followed by a discussion of the factors affecting the choice of providers, methods for developing an appropriate staffing plan and recruitment techniques.

Health Personnel Public Policy

In response to the growing public concern over the shortage of physicians, the federal government invested large sums of money in various health personnel programs. Some states also have supported such programs. These programs were designed to increase the number of health professionals, especially physicians, and improve their distribution by specialty and geographic location.

Federally-Funded Health Personnel Programs

Between 1963 and 1976, federally-funded personnel development programs concentrated on the construction of new medical schools and the expansion of existing schools. Capitation support was linked to enrollment expansion. This approach recognized the shortage of physicians and assumed that an increase in supply ultimately would influence the distribution of physicians.

By 1976, however, greater federal emphasis was being placed on training primary care specialists. Financing was available for developing and expanding residency programs in general internal medicine, general pediatrics and family practice. This policy sought to counteract the effect of subspecialization on the supply of primary care physicians and increase the number of physicians choosing rural practice. The federal policy changes of 1976 also resulted in support to medical schools and residency programs for the development of clinical rotations to expose students to rural practice.

Loan forgiveness programs were initiated in 1965 and liberalized in 1971. Fully operational by 1973, these programs permitted physicians to write off up to 85 percent of their federal loan debt for medical education if they established practices in designated shortage areas.

Grant funds for developing nurse practitioner/physician assistant (NP/PA) training programs also have been made available. These professionals were viewed as a potential alternative for areas experiencing difficulty in recruiting and supporting physicians or as a resource for increasing the capacity of existing physician practices.

Area Health Education Centers (AHECs) were first funded by the Department of Health, Education and Welfare in 1972 to develop support systems that would reduce the problem of professional isolation in rural practice. Funds were applied to continuing education programs, consultation clinics and NP/PA training and practice programs.

The National Health Service Corps (NHSC) was initiated in 1970 to provide scholarships to health professions students, mostly physicians, in exchange for practice in a designated shortage area upon completion of their education. These professionals typically are assigned to sites sponsored by nonprofit community corporations and serve one year for each year of scholarship assistance, with a minimum of two years of service.

These federal health personnel policies have had a significant effect on personnel supply. A 1980 report from the Graduate Medical Education National Advisory Committee (GMENAC) predicted a surplus of physicians by 1990 and recommended a shift in federal support from supply-oriented strategies toward programs aimed at improving the specialty mix of physicians (GMENAC, 1980).

Progress also has been made in altering the mix of primary care versus subspecialty physicians. The Health Professions Educational Assistance Act of 1976 (P.L. 94-484) sought a 50-percent increase in the number of first-year residency positions in primary care (that is, general internal medicine, pediatrics and family practice) by 1979, a goal that was exceeded in 1977 (Jacoby, 1979). While some rural areas have benefited from this shift toward primary care training, the change in geographic distribution of physicians has not been significant. The physician per 100,000 population ratio for all counties increased from 120.3 in 1963 to 137.4 in 1976; for nonmetropolitan counties, the increase was from 73.8 to 74.4 (GMENAC, 1980).

Family practice residency programs have been the most successful in attracting new physicians to rural practice (General Accounting Office, 1978) and some have made a special effort to orient residents to rural practice. Most primary care residency programs, however, have not emphasized rural practice and consequently have not prepared physicians for the unique aspects of practicing in rural areas. Evaluation of loan forgiveness and rural preceptorship programs suggests that they do not significantly influence physician choice of practice location (General Accounting Office, 1978; Lewis and others, 1976). Most physicians who have elected rural rotations or exercised loan forgiveness options already were predisposed to rural practice. However, these programs may be important reinforcements for those considering rural practice.

The success of the National Health Service Corps has been more difficult to evaluate (General Accounting Office, 1978). Many sites have been developed and staffed with NHSC assignees while others eligible for placement of assignees have been unable to attract them. Retention rates of NHSC personnel also have been lower than expected. Recruitment and retention problems often are related to such organizational difficulties as poor planning in the development stage, poor management of the practice site and conflict with community boards. Given the anticipated surplus of physicians in the next decade, it is likely that the NHSC will be reduced drastically over the next few years and therefore will be a decreased source for rural community physician recruitment.

State-Funded Health Personnel Programs

Several states have developed health personnel programs, including support for family practice residencies, scholarship programs for medical students and state-supported recruitment services. One of the most successful state efforts in medical education is the Washington-Alaska-Montana-Idaho program sponsored by the University of Washington Medical School. This program has successfully guided students toward primary care and rural practice through decentralized education that provides early and continuing exposure to rural practice. The state of North Carolina operates a successful physician recruitment program as part of its Office of Rural Health Services, which organizes rural health centers staffed by NP/PAs, provides technical assistance to rural group practices and coordinates placement of NHSC assignees. The continuation of state efforts such as these depends, in part, on state budgetary trends. Some state rural health programs already have been cut while others with demonstrated success probably will continue to receive some state support.

Using Federal and State Programs

Communities and institutions developing rural health services must be thoroughly familiar with the various federal and state personnel programs, since they can be of value in recruiting health professionals. For example, some communities in federally-designated shortage areas may be eligible for NHSC assignees or for loan forgiveness options; some may want to offer sites for rural preceptorships and residency training; others may want to use state-funded recruitment services. The experience of many rural health programs suggests, however, that administrators and community leaders cannot rely totally on federal and state programs to bring health professionals into their communities; local efforts are required as well. Many federal and state programs are staffed by people who are unaware of the needs of particular communities and therefore cannot adequately advocate for resources to address those needs. Many policy makers believe that the increase in supply eventually will solve the personnel problem for some rural areas. However, this does not diminish the need for an organized and informed recruitment effort at the local level to attract physicians and other health professionals best suited to the needs of a particular community.

Types of Health Care Professionals

Many rural communities perceive a need for medical care, but these perceptions are more often based on unanalyzed statements of wants than on a careful assessment of actual need. Few have considered carefully what type of health professionals can best meet the community's needs (whether perceived or actual).

Two organizational variables will influence the choice of providers: size of practice (that is, number of providers) and scope of practice (that is, types of patients seen and levels of care provided). Some communities are too small to support any type of practice. For them, collaboration with other, larger communities may be more appropriate. Some communities are too small to support a full-time physician practice. For them, a nurse practitioner or physician assistant (NP/PA) practice may be more appropriate. Since most physicians prefer to practice with at least one other physician, communities unable to support at least two physicians also should consider the NP/PA alternative.

Regardless of practice size, a rural primary care center must provide a defined range of services, which usually includes acute care, chronic disease maintenance and preventive services for both children and adults, routine gynecological and obstetrical services and some minor surgery. Primary care practices also must have established links with secondary levels of care. In some cases, the range of services provided on-site or by center providers can be fairly narrow if other services are available by referral. For example, a primary care center need not have physicians who provide inpatient services directly if physicians with privileges at a hospital within the service area will accept referrals for hospitalization. Similarly, a center need not provide obstetrical services if physicians providing such services are located within 30 to 60 minutes of the center and will accept referrals. If these services are not readily available by referral, a center must recruit providers who can render a broad range of services and admit and monitor patients requiring hospitalization.

Rural primary care centers typically will be considering five health care personnel categories: physicians; nurse practitioners and physician assistants; support personnel; administrators; and volunteers.

Physicians

When recruiting physicians, administrators must understand the extent to which physician training varies from program to program.

For example, some internal medicine residency programs emphasize general medicine and even prepare physicians to provide some care outside their specialty. Other programs offer only a secondary care emphasis, which may not be appropriate for the primary care needs of rural areas. Similarly, some pediatric residencies emphasize the routine care of children while others are more highly specialized. Within family practice residency training programs, there are variations in emphasis on hospital care, obstetrics and surgery. Administrators therefore must explore the practice expectations of physicians in light of their training and ensure that these expectations match community needs.

Some physicians may be interested in a rural health center position before completing a full residency or internship program. However, hiring these physicians can present problems for rural health centers. First, their clinical training will have been more limited than that of board-eligible physicians, and they are likely to feel less secure in a rural practice with limited technological resources and fewer opportunities for peer consultation. Second, some hospitals will not grant privileges or will grant only limited privileges to physicians without residency training. Finally, experience suggests that the retention rate for such physicians is typically low; they may leave the practice at some point to finish their education or they may have taken the position only as an interim step following internship to explore options before deciding on a residency choice. Although many rural health centers have had positive experiences with these physicians, administrators should be aware of the potential problems before hiring physicians who have not completed residency training.

Even when physicians' training prepares them for the medical needs of a rural community, they may not be prepared for a rural environment. Medical education typically takes place in a large teaching hospital with resources, case mixes and role models that are far removed from the realities of rural practice. Many physicians entering rural practice complain that they are poorly prepared to deal with the primary care needs of their patients because they were trained in settings where patients presented complicated problems and where highly sophisticated diagnostic and treatment technologies were used. Physicians who have received part of their training in rural settings, including practice in small, rural hospitals, are better able to cope with a rural practice than are those whose entire training took place at a university medical center. Those without previous rural experience may need assistance in making the transition to rural practice. This might be accomplished through contact with an Area Health Education Center or a nearby medical school or even through a brief preceptorship with a rural physician.

Physician training programs also rarely prepare them for working in a primary care center with an administrator and a board of directors. Most physicians are unfamiliar with center policy-formation and decision-making processes and many fail to consider these issues when interviewing for a position. Administrators and/or boards therefore must clarify the role of physicians in the center's policy and management processes when interviewing physician candidates.

Primary care services can be provided by internists, pediatricians, obstetrician-gynecologists and family practitioners. Size of practice is the key determinant in choosing between family practitioners and other primary care specialists. It is not surprising that most of the physician-staffed sites in the case studies use family practitioners because these sites are fairly small (two to three physicians). Family practice physicians can treat all ages and provide all aspects of primary care and therefore can practice with a smaller population base. This makes family practice physicians especially well-suited for many rural areas.

In a small, rural practice, there may be limitations to using other primary care specialists. For example, consider a two-physician rural practice with an internist and a pediatrician where the age distribution of the service population generates a greater demand for adult care than pediatrics, which is typical in rural areas. To share the caseload equitably, the pediatrician may be required to treat some adults. When one physician covers for the other after hours or during vacations, he or she must see all patients. Although some internists and pediatricians can and will practice outside their specialties, which this type of practice requires, many prefer not to. Recruiting primary care specialists other than family practitioners for small rural practices may be difficult for this reason.

The need for obstetrical services presents a special problem. Many rural areas may have a greater need for obstetrical (OB) services than for any other primary care service. A high infant mortality rate is often indicative of such a need. Yet many rural health programs fail to plan for the provision of OB services even though the availability of these services constitutes an excellent way to attract both mothers and children as patients. Not all centers can provide these services. A center located more than 30 minutes from a hospital probably will not be able to provide OB services since the physician cannot be readily available for deliveries.

Most rural health centers are too small to efficiently use a full-time obstetrician-gynecologist. Centers staffed by internists and pediatricians may be able to provide routine gynecological services and perhaps pre-natal and post-partum care but must rely on referral arrangements for more specialized gynecological care and deliveries. In many cases, internists will not include OB/GYN services in their practices. Family practitioners usually are trained to provide routine OB/GYN services, but may elect not to handle deliveries for a variety of reasons, among them a desire to avoid late-night calls, concern that the number of deliveries will be insufficient to maintain their skills, concern over the lack of resources for handling high-risk cases or Cesarean section deliveries, concern about the increased malpractice premiums associated with an OB practice or the inability to obtain hospital privileges for obstetrics. If a rural area needs obstetric services, administrators must consider these issues when recruiting physicians and must discuss both center and physician expectations with prospective candidates.

Some rural communities depend on residency programs to staff their centers (as in the Lutheran Hospital case study). Residency programs often are eager to expose their physicians to rural practice and welcome the opportunity to provide a rural rotation. The obvious advantages to the community are a ready source of physicians and possible administrative support from the teaching facility. However, this staffing approach may entail several problems. First, patients may not want to be treated by physicians in training, and they may resent the continual change in physicians associated with residency programs. Second, continuity of care can be jeopardized by the regular turnover of providers. Coordination of services and consistency of administrative procedures can be more difficult to achieve under this kind of arrangement. Third, the residents must be supervised, which requires a faculty commitment to the rural center. Some centers hire a full-time medical director to provide supervision and to assure continuity and consistency; other centers use rotating faculty for supervision and depend upon the center's administrative staff to achieve continuity. These factors must be considered and balanced when communities choose to participate in a residency program.

When recruiting physicians, rural communities tend to assume that any physician will do. However, as the previous discussion suggests, recruitment efforts must be directed toward physicians whose training and expectations best match the size and scope of the planned practice. Consideration should be given to any special needs within the service area, such as a high incidence of a particular chronic disease or occupational health problems. Targeted recruitment efforts can increase the center's ability to meet the particular needs of its service area and improve the chances for recruiting physicians who will be satisfied with the type of practice offered by that center.

Nurse Practitioners and Physician Assistants

Recruiting a full-time physician may not be feasible for many communities. For these communities, a rural health center staffed by a nurse practitioner (NP) or physician assistant (PA) may be an appropriate alternative (as in the Cape Meares and Tehama County case studies). Research on NP/PA deployment suggests that these providers often are placed in rural practices (System Sciences, 1976) and can be easier to recruit and support in a small practice. Size of practice and relative availability of NP/PAs should not be the only considerations in choosing these types of providers, however. There are several legal and reimbursement issues associated with NP/PA practice that typically are beyond administrative control. Other problems result from a misunderstanding of NP/PA roles and their potential contribution to a practice.

The nurse practitioner concept is an expansion of the traditional nursing role. All NPs are registered nurses who receive three to eighteen months of additional training in diagnosis and treatment. Diploma and associate degree nurses attend certificate NP programs, while baccalaureate nurses attend master's programs. Nurse practitioner programs can be affiliated with nursing schools or medical schools or both and tend to emphasize counseling, education and preventive services in addition to diagnostic and treatment skills. These programs train nurses as specialists (such as adult medicine, pediatrics and nurse-midwives) or as generalists (such as family nurse practitioners). National certification procedures have been established for nurse practitioners based on competency exams and training requirements, and many states have their own certification programs for various types of nurse practitioners.

The physician assistant idea emerged in the 1960s when military corpsmen returned from Vietnam with medical skills not readily transferable to the job market. Programs designed to build on those skills by training primary care assistants were among the first PA programs in the country. Students without previous medical training later were accepted into PA programs. As with NP programs, PA programs vary substantially in length of training and admission requirements. Most PA programs are associated with medical schools, extend from one to two academic years and train either specialists or generalists. Several national organizations use exams and training requirements to certify that PAs have specific skills and qualifications.

The legal status of nurse practitioners and physician assistants varies from state to state since licensure is a state responsibility. Nurse practitioners usually are regulated by the state board of nursing. Two general legislative mechanisms—an "additional acts amendment" to nurse practice acts and a "delegatory amendment" to medical practice acts—have been used to define expanded nursing roles. Many states have passed an "additional acts amendment" to their nurse practice act. This amendment defines the tasks a nurse can assume beyond the traditional definition of nursing and typically outlines training requirements, practice settings and relationships to physicians. Other states have passed a "delegatory amendment" to their medical practice act, which permits physicians to delegate certain tasks to nurses. Even in states with an additional acts amendment, it is important to consider the medical practice laws when evaluating the legal status of nurse practitioners. For example, even if the nurse practice act is conducive to NP practice, the medical practice act may restrict physicians who provide back-up for nurse practitioners (Miller and Byrne, 1978).

Physician assistants, representing a new profession with no established regulatory authority, generally come under the aegis of the state board of medicine. Many states have specific PA statutes that define PA roles, training requirements and physician supervision requirements. Some states require both the PA and the supervising physician to register with the state regulatory board (Miller and Byrne, 1978).

Given their training, NP/PAs can play two different roles within a practice. They can serve as physician-substitutes or as physician complements. In a solo NP/PA practice with off-site physician support, NP/PAs serve as the physician-substitute, or primary provider, and refer patients to a physician for consultation and/or hospitalization. This role emphasizes their ability to diagnose and treat common illnesses, manage chronic diseases and provide preventive services. Research on task delegation suggests that nurse practitioners and physician assistants can manage up to 70 percent of all patient care needs at the primary care level (Robin and Spector, 1980), making this an effective mechanism for a physician practice as well. In the latter instance, the NP/PA can work jointly with the physician to manage routine patient problems, or the NP/PA can manage the preliminary aspects of patient exams while the physician completes the diagnosis and treatment process.

The physician-complement model emphasizes NP/PA skills in areas not generally associated with physician practice, such as counseling and education. Under this arrangement, the physician as primary provider refers patients to the NP/PA for counseling or patient teaching services. The complementary role is not amenable to a solo NP/PA practice where acute and chronic care are paramount; nor is this role always appropriate for an NP/PA-physician joint practice if the NP/PA is needed to increase the physician's capacity to meet patients' basic medical needs.

Administrators must be aware of state law pertaining to nurse practitioners and physician assistants to ensure that their roles at a center are legal. They must examine training and supervisory requirements, prohibited acts, restrictions on practice settings and rules governing prescription writing and dispensing. Both administrators and physicians must clearly define the NP/PA role before recruiting these providers. One study found that 44 percent of all nurse practitioners who changed jobs after graduation did so because they were unable to use their skills in the job situation (Report of the Physician Extender Workgroup, 1977). Job descriptions should outline the scope of services to be provided and define the relationships between NP/PAs and back-up physicians and administration. The expectations and skills of prospective candidates can be matched with center needs only if these needs are clearly articulated in advance. The Hemmingford case study illustrates the problems that can arise when NP/PA roles are not defined prior to recruitment.

Three other important issues are associated with the employment of nurse practitioners and physician assistants: (1) reimbursement policies; (2) patient acceptance; and (3) quality of care.

Reimbursement

While most states have addressed or are addressing the legal status of NP/PAs, recognizing them as reimbursable providers has been a slower process. Until passage of the Rural Health Clinic Services Act of 1977 (P.L. 95-210), Medicare reimbursement for NP/PA services was illegal while Medicaid reimbursement varied from state to state. With passage of P.L. 95-210, the federal government recognized NP/PA services as reimbursable under certain circumstances. Specifically, the law provides for reimbursement on a reasonable cost basis under both Medicare and Medicaid if the services are provided within a rural health clinic in an underserved area. States must certify sites for reimbursement if the state has enacted legislation governing NP/PA practice and if it permits NP/PA practice without full-time physician back-up. The definition of rural health clinic is sufficiently broad to include private practice settings. However, the reasonable cost reimbursement method applied to health centers differs from that used for physicians in private practice. (Private physicians usually are reimbursed on a fee-for-service basis using usual and customary charge schedules.) The reporting requirements associated with cost-based payment make this a fairly complicated reimbursement mechanism for most small rural centers to manage.

Rural centers not meeting federal certification requirements cannot bill Medicare for NP/PA services. Medicaid policy varies from state to state, as do the policies of other third-party payers. Many third parties have not explicitly addressed the issue of NP/PA reimbursement, others recognize that physicians are billing for these services under their own names and have accepted this practice, while others specifically deny payment when a service is provided by a practitioner other than a physician (Miller and Byrne, 1978).

Patient Acceptance

The concept of a nurse practitioner or physician assistant is new to most patients. Research on patient acceptance of these providers demonstrates that the physician is a key figure (Litman, 1977). Patient acceptance is high if the physician introduces the NP/PA to patients (see the Tehama County case study). Acceptance is less likely when physician support is ambivalent or absent. Rural health centers staffed by NP/PAs should conduct community education efforts to familiarize potential patients with the NP/PA role as it is defined for the center.

Quality of Care

Several studies have examined the quality of care provided by NP/PAs. The findings suggest that, within the appropriate scope of practice, NP/PA care usually is equal to or better than that provided by physicians (Ott, 1976; Levine and others, 1976; Runyan, 1975).

Successful use of NP/PAs depends on careful role definition, compliance with licensure requirements, consideration of reimbursement issues and a well-defined relationship between the NP/PA and the supervising physician. Although it is often assumed that NP/PAs are not as concerned as physicians about issues of professional isolation, continuing education and consultation, experience indicates that these are key concerns for mid-level practitioners. Administrators failing to recognize these concerns may have difficulty recruiting and retaining NP/PAs.

Support Personnel

The number and type of support personnel employed by a rural health center vary with size of practice. Primary care practices usually require two to three support staff per full-time physician. A larger practice may be able to use support personnel with specialty training, such as laboratory technicians or medical secretaries. Smaller sites typically cannot recruit such personnel and require fewer staff with more flexibly defined roles. These practices usually combine medical assistant and laboratory functions into one job. Similarly, reception and medical records activities can be combined.

In some communities, it may be possible to recruit personnel with previous experience in a medical practice. For example, licensed practical nurses with hospital experience can be trained in office procedures and lab work. Community members without previous medical experience or training can be given on-the-job training in basic clinical and clerical procedures. However, on-the-job training must be carefully planned and regularly evaluated. While many support tasks can be taught, administrators should not assume that providers are prepared to plan the appropriate training and evaluate it. State laws governing the performance of tasks by unlicensed personnel also must be taken into consideration.

Administrators

Every center, regardless of size, must routinely perform a variety of administrative tasks, including personnel management, planning, financial management, and community and board relations. Grant-supported centers also must manage their grants, monitor compliance with regulations and maintain relationships with the grant agency. Administrative arrangements will vary from center to center depending on center sponsorship (the organization legally responsible for the center) and center size. Centers with ties to larger institutions, such as a hospital or medical school, may limit their on-site administrative functions to billing, bookkeeping and day-to-day supervision (see the University Medical Center case study), while planning, financial management and community relations may be the responsibility of the sponsoring organization. This arrangement provides access to administrative support services often not available in rural areas. At the same time, however, center administration may be low on the sponsoring organization's list of priorities, leading to delays in addressing problems. Off-site administration also makes the center dependent on the sponsoring organization and reduces its potential for developing local administrative capabilities.

Freestanding centers need to develop their own on-site administrative capabilities by using full- or part-time administrators or assigning certain management functions to providers. While many centers cannot justify full-time managers, part-time administrators can be difficult to recruit since people with administrative experience and training typically seek full-time employment. Full-time administrators, however, can assume many responsibilities crucial to center survival, including staff recruitment. Trained health administrators may be as difficult to attract to rural areas as are physicians. Some graduate programs in health administration now prepare students for careers in rural health management, and graduates of these programs will be most interested in positions with a broad range of responsibilities and authority.

Many communities seek out individuals with administrative or business management experience outside the health care field; others recruit individuals experienced in writing grant proposals and fund raising (see the Hemmingford case study). These managers can function effectively as center administrators if training opportunities exist to expose them to the unique aspects of health care administration. The Hemmingford administrator, for example, engages in a self-education program by visiting other sites. This may be a necessary step for managers lacking previous experience or training in health care administration.

Delegating management responsibilities to providers often poses a special problem. Few providers are trained or experienced in management or proposal-writing techniques. Providers may not be able to balance their dual responsibilities for patient care and management (see the Cape Meares case study). In most instances, management will be low on the list of provider priorities. Providers may be better able to assume management responsibilities if the center is small and follows a traditional private practice model. Support personnel, preferably with previous medical practice experience, still will be needed to perform bookkeeping and billing functions. Several consulting firms also specialize in practice management and can assist a provider-managed center in establishing administrative procedures and monitoring practice performance.

Volunteers

Many rural health centers are attracted to the idea of using community volunteers, since it symbolizes community involvement and support and provides a source of free labor. In fact, before widespread funding was available in the mid-1970s, many centers used volunteers as the mainstay of their operations. When funding became available and full-time employees could be hired, many of these centers experienced difficulty in making the transition from a volunteer-based to a more formal employee-based organization (see the Cape Meares case study).

Several important management issues arise when considering the use of volunteers. First, because volunteers need training and supervision, a full-time staff member should be assigned this task. Second, problems with accountability, reliability, liability and patient privacy must be anticipated before a volunteer staff is used. And third, the use of volunteers may affect the center's image in the community. As many case studies in this book suggest, rural centers are often perceived as free clinics, and the use of volunteers can contribute to this misconception. These trade-offs must be carefully evaluated before volunteers are included in a staffing plan.

The Staffing Plan

Problems with overstaffing and/or the hiring of inappropriate types of providers can be avoided by developing a staffing plan after a careful analysis of anticipated demand for service. Various measures of need are used to project patient volume. Federal designations of underservice represent one measure. A Critical Manpower Shortage Area is defined by the physician-to-population ratio. The designation Medically Underserved Area incorporates this ratio and other measures of need, such as the infant mortality rate and the percentage of the population over 65 or under the poverty level. Additional measures of need include the number of practices in the area closed to Medicaid or Medicare patients, waiting time for appointments, travel time to existing resources or evidence of community support based on surveys.

Many health centers use these indicators in projecting their demand for services, but experience suggests that these indicators may produce service projections that far exceed actual demand. This happens for several reasons. First, consumer perceptions of the need for services typically differ from the normative standards established by health professionals (Aday and Anderson, 1975). Second, many people in underserved rural areas already have established sources of care (Aday and Anderson, 1975). The provider may be located at a distance and used only for acute conditions, but the relationship persists and may be firmly established. Consumers generally are reluctant to sever these existing relationships in favor of new service opportunities closer to home, especially if the new services are perceived as potentially unstable. Centers experiencing a constant turnover of providers are especially vulnerable to this perception and will find it difficult to effect a consumer shift in loyalty.

Because of discrepancies between need and demand, many centers tend to overestimate utilization if they use measures of need in the planning stage, a situation which leads to overstaffing. Many do not plan for phasing-in professional and support staff—starting small and growing as needed. Often, the receipt of grant support fosters this tendency to begin an overly large program with too many providers. Centers must rank their needs and evaluate the feasibility of meeting each one. Once priorities are set, the center can gradually add services and staff as initial services become established and used.

Developing the Plan

Centers can develop realistic staffing plans by following a three-step procedure.

Defining the Service Area

All staffing plans begin with a careful and realistic definition of the service area. Adjustments must be made for geographic barriers that might inhibit the use of a particular site. Local trade patterns, including shopping habits, also will affect the service area. People may have loyalties to a particular hospital and avoid a center that uses another hospital for secondary care. County boundaries also can inhibit travel patterns and hence center utilization. These and other geographic, social and political factors must be accounted for in defining the service area.

Estimating Demand

Once the service area has been defined, census data can be correlated with data from the National Ambulatory Care Survey (available from the National Center for Health Statistics), which reports actual utilization of ambulatory care services by age, sex and race. These data will help produce more accurate estimates of utilization than those produced by a need analysis, especially if regional data from the survey are used. Some adaptations may be required if characteristics of the local population vary significantly from those of the population of the region. If local utilization data are not available, adjustments for local differences must be based on estimates and realistic expectations.

Visit projections resulting from a correlation of census and National Ambulatory Care Survey data are based on a 100-percent penetration of the market. Since no center can expect to capture an entire market, the market share must be estimated. This estimate will be conditioned by local factors. For example, if the population is fairly mobile and exhibits high migration rates, or if the population is increasing, market penetration should be high since families new to an area are more likely to use new services (Hays and Leaman, 1976). Market penetration also can be expected to be high if the service area recently lost a physician and new relationships have not been formed

(Wollack and Kretz, 1979). It also may be high if the service population is familiar with the practice model; for example, a family practice staffed by a physician rather than a primary care center staffed by a nurse practitioner or physician assistant.

Estimating Provider Productivity

The demand estimate derived in Step 2 then is correlated with provider productivity to estimate the number of providers needed by the practice. The American Medical Association publishes an annual *Profile of Medical Practice,* which includes data on the number of visits per physician by specialty. This can be used to estimate physician productivity and make adjustments for differences in productivity among specialties. Other adjustments may be necessary, however. For example, physicians who recently have completed their residency generally see fewer patients than do physicians who have practiced for years. The use of residents therefore can be expected to limit productivity. Hospital care provided by center physicians also will affect productivity since time spent on hospital rounds is a necessary part of a hospital practice. (As discussed later in this chapter, the benefits of a hospital practice may outweigh any reductions in center productivity.) Finally, new centers typically experience lower productivity regardless of the type of providers used because all patients are new and require more time as providers establish data bases for continuing care and become familiar with their patients.

Productivity estimates for nurse practitioners and physician assistants (NP/PAs) may be more difficult to derive since these estimates will be affected by their role. When serving as primary providers, NP/PAs can usually see between 15 and 25 patients per day (Brooks and others, 1979). When practicing with a physician, their productivity will depend on the practice arrangement. For example, overall productivity will be lower if all patients see both the physician and the NP/PA during a visit (Glenn and Goldman, 1976).

Realistic estimates of provider productivity are important for two reasons: (1) to help plan for facility size and staffing during the center's developmental stage; and (2) to avoid disputes over productivity that can arise once the center is operational. (The Hemmingford case study illustrates this problem.) Ideally, expectations for provider productivity should be defined before providers are recruited and should be discussed with applicants. Health professional training generally does not familiarize providers with productivity levels or prepare them to discuss the issue with prospective employers. These issues must be discussed during recruitment to determine whether community or administration expectations match those of the providers being recruited. Unless this issue is resolved, it can become a source of tension between providers and boards or administrators, especially if providers are recent graduates, who tend to see fewer patients per hour, use fewer prescriptions and hospitalize less often than do older physicians. Conflicts arise when board members and administrators expect new physicians to have the same practice style as the older physicians who once served the community.

Finding reliable provider productivity measures is a continuing dilemma for health care managers. The most common measure is the patient visit, but it is important to recognize that numerous factors affect its usefulness. For example, the length of visits will vary because new patients typically need longer visits than do return patients. Length of visit also varies by diagnosis. These factors often account for the variation in productivity across physician specialties and illustrate the difficulty associated with comparing physician productivity only on the basis of number of patient visits. To compensate for these factors, it is advisable to calculate productivity by visit type and/or diagnosis.

These factors also must be considered when using patient visits to determine the relative productivity of nurse practitioners and physician assistants (NP/PAs) versus physicians. In some practices, NP/PAs handle routine problems and refer complicated cases to the physician, which means their productivity will be higher than that of the physician. In other situations, the physician handles most medical problems and refers patients requiring extensive health counseling or education to the NP/PA, resulting in higher productivity rates for the physician. Administrators must be sensitive to the factors influencing the accuracy of patient visits as a measure of productivity if they are to fairly assess the contribution each provider makes to a practice.

Low provider productivity often is cited as the reason for a center's inability to achieve financial self-sufficiency. In some cases, providers are unaware of their own productivity rates and the effect productivity has on center viability. A good management information system that provides monthly data on visits by provider enables continuous feedback to providers on performance measures. Administrators also should establish close working relationships with providers to facilitate discussions of provider performance issues that are affecting center viability, such as scheduling of patients, utilization of provider time on recordkeeping or administrative matters and provider attitudes toward charges for services. The situation cited in the Hemmingford case study, for example, could have been improved by this kind of ongoing dialogue.

A center's inability to achieve financial self-sufficiency also can stem from an insufficient demand for services, low fee schedules, ineffective collection procedures, billing inefficiencies and abnormally high overhead costs. Providers cannot be expected to compensate in volume for deficiencies in administrative procedures or demand for services. All potential causes for financial problems should be carefully analyzed before providers are asked to change practice styles and increase patient volume. Conflicts often can be avoided if providers and administrators work together in establishing realistic goals that recognize both provider capabilities and center needs.

Staffing Pattern Variations

Center staffing patterns are initially conditioned by the size of practice that can reasonably be supported. If the service area can support only a single physician or NP/PA, certain problems will be created for both the provider and consumers. First, a solo provider cannot be on-call every day of the year and every minute of the day. If arrangements for after-hours coverage cannot be made, and if the center is essentially a nine-to-five operation, many prospective patients will turn to other resources with better coverage capabilities. Second, a solo practice may not be able to provide hospital care since daily hospital rounds would leave the office unstaffed. This situation may affect utilization and also make the center unattractive to physicians, since they often view practices without an inpatient component as unsatisfying. Continuity of care also may be jeopardized if the inpatient and outpatient components of care are not managed by the same provider. Finally, the inability to provide hospital care also will mean loss of a potential revenue source that can be essential to long-range viability (Wollack and Kretz, 1979).

Because of these and other problems with coverage and hospital care capabilities, small centers unable to support two or more providers may find it difficult to attract not only providers but also patients. One alternative is to locate at a site that is outside the community itself but readily accessible in order to draw from a larger population base and thereby support a larger practice. Another alternative is to work with other communities in establishing a network (similar to that discussed in the C. T. Meyer Hospital case study).

In some cases, a physician and nurse practitioner/physician assistant combination may be financially feasible and make the site more attractive to providers because of the opportunity for consultation and coverage. Under this arrangement, the NP/PA practices with the physician in the office and covers the practice when the physician is at the hospital. Provisions still must be made for physician coverage during vacations and after hours and for patient hospitalizations during those times.

Centers must develop flexible staffing patterns and adapt to changes in utilization trends and needs. In general, it is easier to expand as the need arises than to initiate personnel reductions because of overstaffing situations. One approach is to establish a standard for new appointments (for example, specifying that new patients should wait no more than one or two weeks for an appointment). Once the waiting period begins to exceed this standard and continues to do so over a set time period (a number of months), an additional provider may be needed. When a decision is reached to add a new provider, the center must consider the implications for adding support personnel. For example, some functions can be performed with the same number of personnel, while others will require additional personnel. Because an additional provider may also create new space requirements, recruitment efforts should be coordinated with any facility expansion needs.

Management needs also change as centers expand, and new administrative problems, especially in coordination, will emerge. Changes in administration also can be disruptive; for example, as a center changes from the provider-manager to the full-time administrator model, or from a part-time to a full-time administrator model. (Consider the transition problems discussed in the Cape Meares case study.) These changes must be anticipated, planned for and fully explained to the staff. Job descriptions should be rewritten and discussed with center staff members so that all changes in authority and responsibility are clearly understood.

Changes in staffing patterns always carry the potential for operational disruption. New providers bring their own ideas about practice organization and style and will attempt to change certain center procedures to match their ideas. The best solution is to accommodate their ideas without significantly changing the organization of the center (rather than changing center procedures to fit the provider, which is often the case). Disruption and unnecessary center changes can be avoided by discussing provider expectations for practice arrangements during the recruitment process to ensure that the goals of both the provider and the organization are in agreement. Some compromising by both parties may be necessary. Balancing the new provider's need for a feeling of investment in the organization with the need for organizational consistency and stability is a difficult but crucial task for the administrator.

Recruitment and Retention

Recruiting and retaining qualified providers presents special problems for rural communities. Several factors influence physician decisions about practice location, and these factors will influence the way physicians should be recruited. Many of these same factors also influence NP/PAs and will similarly affect efforts to recruit them. Recruitment techniques must be carefully planned and implemented. Several strategies are available, but the selection of strategy must be made with care and be appropriate to the community and its special needs.

Physician Recruitment

While research points to a number of factors that influence a physician's choice of practice location, eight appear to be the most significant (Cooper and others, 1975; Evashwick, 1976).

☐ *Background of the Physician.* Physicians raised in a rural setting are more likely to select rural practices.

☐ *Opportunities for Partnership or Group Practice.* Physicians today are less likely to select solo practices given their coverage and consultation limitations.

☐ *Place of Medical Training.* Physicians trained in medical schools and/or residency programs in or near rural areas are more likely to choose rural practices. Also, physicians trained in state-supported medical schools are more likely to choose rural practice than are those trained in private medical schools.

☐ *Availability of Clinical Support Personnel.* Physicians are concerned about the availability of qualified support staff, especially nurses.

☐ *Opportunities for Continuing Education and Consultation with Other Physicians.* Most physicians, and especially new physicians, are concerned about maintaining their skills and avoiding professional isolation. Access to peers through continuing education and consultation opportunities therefore can be important.

☐ *Opportunities for a Hospital Practice.* Hospital practice is an integral part of medical education and most physicians expect to have a hospital practice.

☐ *Arrangements for After-Hours Coverage.* Physicians are no longer willing to be, nor should they be, constantly on-call. At the same time, they are anxious to ensure adequate coverage for their patients.

☐ *Needs of Spouse and Family.* Even if physicians find a practice arrangement professionally satisfying, they are unlikely to choose that practice if the community cannot meet their family needs.

Rural communities must consider these factors when developing a recruitment strategy. Five of these factors are associated with organizational design, suggesting that organizational issues are as important as geographic location. As the National Health Service Corps experience demonstrates, rural communities probably will not be successful in attracting physicians who are not receptive to rural living. At the same time, a rural community cannot realistically expect to attract physicians if the practice arrangement fails to match the expectations of most physicians. Community leaders or administrators responsible for recruitment should visit other communities that have successfully recruited physicians and should consult with program directors in residency programs to learn more about physician expectations about rural practices. Recruitment efforts will be more successful if communities anticipate physician needs for support personnel, group practice arrangements, hospital practice, coverage, continuing education and consultation.

Rural communities also must offer competitive compensation packages. Some physicians will find a straight salary arrangement attractive to avoid concern with the financial impact of their practice decisions, and others will seek incentive systems that reward them for productivity. Given the problems many centers have encountered with productivity, it is advisable for centers to provide some form of incentive system in their compensation plans. Hiring a physician on a fee-for-service basis, however, also can be problematic, since the absence of a guaranteed caseload or a service population economically able to support a physician practice places the physician at considerable risk.

Several options are available for balancing the need for guarantees to attract physicians with the need for productivity. Physicians can be guaranteed a salary for the first two to three years while they establish a caseload, after which their incomes would be derived solely based on productivity. Another option is to combine a base salary with productivity incentives. For example, physicians would receive a guaranteed salary regardless of productivity plus a percentage of the revenue generated by the practice; or they would receive a guaranteed salary for a predetermined patient volume plus the revenues generated (less administrative expenses) for all patients exceeding that amount. Whichever arrangement is chosen, the need for productivity must be balanced with adequate time for the patient/physician visit. Any system based solely on productivity may encourage overutilization and could jeopardize the quality of care.

The compensation plan also must take into account revenues generated by a hospital practice. Some centers (as in the Hemmingford case study) allow physicians to retain all hospital revenues and may even assign inpatient billing responsibilities to the physician. This may not be advisable if hospital care is an essential part of the center's service and financial goals. A more appropriate approach, and one used more often, is to make no distinction between hospital and office revenue in determining physician compensation.

A comprehensive fringe benefit package, including such items as health and life insurance, malpractice coverage, medical society dues, vacation and sick time, and time off and reimbursement for continuing education, also will help attract prospective applicants. However, administrators must weigh various alternatives and balance physician needs with those of the center. The attractiveness of each fringe benefit will vary from physician to physician, but income generally is the most important issue. In any event, the compensation plan should be developed in detail before recruitment efforts are initiated, and administrators should be flexible and willing to negotiate.

Nurse Practitioner/Physician Assistant Recruitment

Several of the factors affecting the recruitment of physicians also affect the recruitment of nurse practitioners/physician assistants (NP/PAs), since they also are concerned with issues of coverage, consultation, opportunities for continuing education and practice scope (the types of patients to be seen and services to be provided). Some NP/PAs may want hospital practices, although this is uncommon (most hospitals will not grant NP/PA privileges). They will want to know about their relationships with center physicians and with the community and their roles in management and policy formation. Like physicians, they are equally concerned about lifestyle issues for themselves and for their families. Compensation is also an important issue. While most NP/PAs are hired on a straight salary basis, many centers have developed compensation plans that include productivity incentives. As with physicians, expectations about practice arrangements, coverage, scope of practice and compensation must be discussed and negotiated during recruitment.

Recruitment Techniques

The key to a successful recruitment effort is organization. It is imperative that one individual have overall responsibility for the recruitment effort, even though other people (staff and community) should be involved. Local physicians, especially those from the hospital providing secondary care, should be involved in recruiting both physicians and NP/PAs. New providers will want assurances that they are welcome in the medical community and can consult with and refer to physicians in the area. (In the Montgomery County Hospital case study, for example, the medical staff's opposition to the satellites may be a major factor in the hospital's recruitment problem.) Hospital administrative staff also should offer encouragement for providers seeking admitting privileges. Civic leaders, board members and staff also are essential to helping new providers feel a part of the community and offering evidence of community support for the center and its providers.

Before initiating a recruitment effort, administrators must develop a clear job description for providers and a sample contract. Issues to be addressed include: compensation, fringe benefits, hours, scope of practice, hospital privileges and responsibilities, after-hours coverage, malpractice, continuing education, relationships between physicians and NP/PAs, and the provider's role in management and policy formation. Those involved in the recruitment effort should be familiar with all contract provisions in order to present consistent information. Administrators should determine in advance which aspects of the contract are negotiable and which are not, remembering the importance of being flexible without compromising the basic goals of the center.

Information about the center and the community should be sent to applicants in advance. Positive aspects of work and life in the community should be highlighted. Efforts should be made to identify the particular needs of the applicant's family and address them as well. Recruiters must be honest in responding to legitimate concerns expressed by applicants or their families, since distortions or misrepresentations of living and working environments ultimately will lead to provider dissatisfaction, which in turn may result in high turnover rates, increased recruiting costs and a loss of patients.

Techniques for physician recruitment include the following:

☐ *Advertising.* Advertising in professional journals and the health care section of major newspapers is one way to attract potential candidates. Because these publications usually are circulated nationally, responses will include many physicians who are not good candidates because of their specialty or geographic preference. Advertising is generally viewed by experienced administrators as one of the least productive methods of physician recruitment.

☐ *Recruitment Services.* Several professional firms specialize in recruiting physicians. The fee typically is equal to a portion of the first year's salary if the candidate is employed through the firm's effort. These firms are experienced in recruitment techniques and have a network of contacts generally unavailable to rural communities. Administrators should carefully check the firm's references before contracting for services.

☐ *Contacts with Medical Schools and Residencies.* This is viewed as one of the most successful techniques for physician recruitment, since new graduates are the most likely candidates for a new practice. Establishing relationships with faculty members who can inform residents about available sites can be very beneficial. If a center already has physicians on staff, these physicians can contact their own medical schools and residency programs to help in the recruitment process. Some centers offer rotations for medical students or residents as a method of recruitment. While physicians rotating through the center may not elect to practice at the center, they will make other physicians aware of the center and its practice opportunities.

☐ *State and Medical Society Recruitment Services.* Some state governments and many medical societies offer recruitment assistance. Some provide a list of physicians who have inquired about practice opportunities and who must be contacted by the center itself. Others offer a careful matching service in which center needs are correlated with physician expectations.

☐ *National Health Service Corps (NHSC).* The NHSC helps match providers with communities in designated shortage areas. Because competition for the limited number of Corps assignees is intense, communities should contact Corps-obligated medical students and residents directly and not wait for the Corps to send prospective assignees. Corps physicians considering a variety of placement options can be influenced by personal contacts with particular communities, and communities are the best representatives of what they can offer prospective providers.

Many of the techniques for recruiting physicians can be used to recruit nurse practitioners/physician assistants (NP/PAs), among them advertising in professional journals and newspapers, contacting NP and PA programs, sponsoring student NP/PAs for preceptorships and seeking NHSC assignees. Professional recruitment firms are less helpful since they usually lack experience in dealing with these providers.

Several important factors must be considered in planning a recruitment program for health professionals. First, because no single strategy will meet the needs of every rural area or center, several strategies should be attempted. Second, recruitment is a slow, continual process that must be carefully planned in advance. Recruitment is less effective as a crisis response than as an ongoing management activity. The process itself can take from six months to a year or more. Third, personal contact has proven to be the most effective means of recruitment. Regardless of the strategy used to generate initial prospective candidates, administrators should follow-up using a personalized approach. Fourth, not all applicants are appropriate for rural health center practices. Interested providers should be asked to explain their reasons for considering rural practice, particularly if they are leaving another practice. Fifth, administrators must consider the degree to which the practice styles and philosophies of providers at the center will be compatible. Providers who will be working together should be given an opportunity to meet and discuss their practice plans and styles. Finally, the recruitment process will be compromised if administrative, medical community and public support is not evident.

Retention

Retention issues cannot be isolated from recruitment issues, since professional staff turnover often results from deficiencies in meeting provider needs identified during the recruitment process. Many of the reasons cited by providers for leaving a practice are related to the same issues that make provider recruitment difficult. When a physician or other provider leaves, the center must first determine why. Was it because of a community characteristic that cannot be changed but can be anticipated in recruiting a replacement? Were there organizational problems that could be resolved? Was the provider dissatisfied with the center's compensation package? Did the provider want more leave time, more peer contact, a different patient mix or a greater say in policy making? Administrators should analyze these variables, identify those that are within administrative control and then evaluate the organizational impact of addressing them.

Unfortunately, some centers experience retention problems no matter how carefully they plan and recruit. There are aspects of rural practice and rural living that cannot be changed and may inevitably result in some provider dissatisfaction. In general, Americans have become highly mobile and change jobs frequently; health providers are no exception. Personnel turnover can be a serious problem for rural health center viability. This underscores the importance of evaluating staff turnover trends and making appropriate adjustments.

Conclusions

Predictions of a physician surplus may mislead rural communities in evaluating their recruitment potential. Larger rural communities that already have physicians but need more probably will find it easier to recruit new physicians and replace those who leave practice. Communities with no physicians but able to support two or more also may find it easier to recruit in the future. In fact, some communities already are experiencing the positive effects of the increases in supply and number of primary care physicians.

Despite the predictions, however, some communities may still find it difficult to recruit. Perhaps they are too small to support more than one physician, are located too far from a hospital or cannot offer a living environment attractive to professionals concerned about cultural and social opportunities and community services. Communities considering the nurse practitioner/physician assistant alternative also must assess the impact of a physician surplus on these providers. Much of the public policy support for training and reimbursing NP/PAs has been rooted in the notion of a physician shortage. As this changes, support for mid-level practitioners may change. States may amend their present legislation to restrict NP/PA practice, and states without NP/PA legislation may find it increasingly difficult to enact supportive legislation. Communities looking to these providers must constantly monitor the changing political environment and how it is affecting NP/PA practice.

The predicted surplus will not resolve all the problems associated with recruiting health professionals to rural areas. First, the shortage of certain types of physicians will continue, especially primary care physicians, who are most appropriate for rural practice. The supply of primary care physicians will depend, in part, on whether public financing for their training is continued and at what level. Should public funding be discontinued, the growth rate for primary care physicians will be highly uncertain. As a result, competition for internists, pediatricians and, in particular, family practitioners could intensify. Second, the urban bias inherent in medical education is not likely to abate. Unless there are significant changes in the orientation of physician training, new graduates will be unprepared for rural practice. Finally, even if the surplus market forces more physicians into rural areas, many may establish rural practices only reluctantly. Like many of the physicians in the National Health Service Corps, these physicians will be less satisfied and centers will experience high turnover rates.

Even with an increase in the number of physicians, rural communities must pay careful attention to the type and number of providers they need. Many of the issues discussed in this chapter will continue to be important in a surplus environment if communities are to achieve a match between their needs and those of available providers. The need for community-sponsored rural health centers may diminish if more physicians are attracted into private practice in rural areas. Where the need still exists, careful planning will be required.

Recruitment and retention of competent and productive providers are crucial to the success of rural health delivery systems. Facilities and financial resources are meaningless if physicians and other professionals are not attracted to a practice. For many rural areas, recruitment needs to begin by understanding those changes in medical practice that created the current health professional distribution problem. In some cases, a change in expectations may be the first step in the recruitment process. Community centers must develop realistic organizational designs and staffing patterns, define their expectations for provider productivity and create well-organized recruitment efforts. The health care environment is changing constantly, and public policy changes will affect the success of many rural recruiting efforts. Communities that understand these changes and create flexible plans will have the greatest chance for success in meeting their health care needs.

References

Aday, L.A., and Anderson, R. *Development of Indices of Access to Medical Care*, p. 38. Ann Arbor, MI: Health Administration Press, 1975.

Brooks, E., and others. Rural primary care and new health practitioners. Paper presented at the American Health Planning Association annual meeting, 1979.

Cooper, J.K., and others. Rural or urban practice factors influencing the locational decision of primary care physicians. *Inquiry*, 12(1975):18.

Evashwick, C. The role of group practice in the distribution of physicians in nonmetropolitan areas. *Med. Care*, 14(1976):808.

General Accounting Office. *Progress and Problems in Improving the Availability of*

Primary Care Providers in Underserved Areas. Washington, D.C.: Report to the Congress of the United States by the Comptroller General, 1978.

Glenn, J.K., and Goldman, J. Strategies for productivity with physician extenders. *West. J. Med.,* 124(1976):249.

Graduate Medical Education National Advisory Committee. *GMENAC Summary Report Volume I.* Washington, D.C.: Department of Health and Human Services, 1980.

Hays, P., and Leaman, L. Delivery of health care by satellite: Hospital-based ambulatory care. *Hosp. Health Serv. Adm.,* 21(1976):55.

Jacoby, I. Impact of the Health Professions Educational Assistance Act on specialty distribution among first-year residents. *Public Health Rep.,* 94(1979):104.

Levine, D., and others. The role of new health practitioners in a prepaid group practice: Provider differences in process and outcomes of medical care. *Med. Care,* 14(1976):326.

Lewis, C., and others. *A Right to Health, the Problem of Access to Primary Medical Care.* New York City: John Wiley & Sons, 1976.

Litman, T., Jr. Public perceptions of the physician's assistant: A survey of attitudes and opinions of rural Iowa and Minnesota residents. *Am. J. Public Health,* 62(1977):343.

Miller and Byrne, Inc. *Review and Analysis of State Legislation and Reimbursement Practices of Physician's Assistants and Nurse Practitioners.* Rockville, MD: 1978.

Ott, J. Child health associates stimulated patient study. Paper presented at Ambulatory Pediatrics Association meeting, St. Louis, 1976.

Report of the Physician Extender Workgroup. (77 [HRA] 602-14). Washington, D.C.: U. S. Dept. of Health, Education and Welfare, June 1977.

Robin, D., and Spector, K. Delegation potential of primary care visits by physician assistants, medex and primex. *Med. Care,* 18(1980):1114.

Runyan, J.W., Jr. The Memphis chronic disease program comparison in outcomes and the nurses extended roles. J. AM. MED. ASSN., 231(1975):264.

System Sciences, Inc. *Nurse Practitioner and Physician Assistant Training and Development Study: Executive Summary* (230 [HRA] 75-0198). Washington, D.C.: U. S. Dept. of Health, Education and Welfare, June 1976.

Wollack, S., and Kretz, S. Self-sufficiency in rural medical practices: Obstacles and solutions. Unpublished paper, Brandeis University, Boston, 1979.

4

Financing the Development of Rural Primary Care Centers

Roland Palmer, M.H.A.
Ann Eward, Ph.D.

Mr. Palmer is president of Primary Care Consultants, Inc. and executive vice-president of the Sparta Health Center in Sparta, Michigan.

Dr. Eward is an assistant professor in the Department of Community Health Science, College of Medicine, at Michigan State University, Lansing.

Financing the Development of Rural Primary Care Centers

A major factor contributing to the growth of rural primary care centers during the 1970s was the availability of both public and private financial resources for developing, operating and expanding community-based health centers. Community-based health centers are defined here as centers located in an identifiable community in which community members are actively involved in center activities. They may be sponsored by community corporations, hospitals, public health departments or provider groups. The concepts discussed in this chapter refer to freestanding centers that may be affiliated with a sponsoring organization. In contrast to sponsorship, health centers may be owned and operated by larger entities, in which case they are satellites of the sponsor and operated in a manner consistent with the financial conditions of that organization. Hospital satellites are treated as part of the hospital, and public health satellites are treated as part of the public health department.

During the 1970s, resources for developmental funding included everything from government programs, such as the Rural Health Initiative program (RHI), to privately funded programs, such as the Innovations in Ambulatory Primary Care project (IAPC) supported by the W. K. Kellogg Foundation. Operational funding sources also were expanded during that decade; one example was the Rural Health Clinic Services Act (P.L. 95-210), which was the most notable attempt to alter the traditional pattern of physician-only reimbursement for health care services.

Financial resources, although substantially more available during the 1970s, were not always effectively used by health centers or their sponsoring organizations. By 1980, many health centers supported through external funding agencies were no longer able to continue operating once their developmental subsidies expired, and the financial future for most rural health centers appears tenuous at best.

The purpose of this chapter is two-fold: to offer a strategy for effective resource identification, development and utilization; and to discuss an accompanying strategy for maximizing reimbursement and expanding the resource base.

Developing a Resource Strategy

Resource planning is an integrative strategy for securing funds from a variety of sources. Once a health center has been operating for a period of time, it may generate sufficient patient care dollars to fund its medical services. But new program development and educational activities, as well as allied health services, usually must be subsidized by other funding sources. These may include government programs, foundations and philanthropies, community organizations, hospitals or other health care organizations, and educational institutions. While for-profit organizations would seek investors for new program development or diversification ventures, nonprofit health centers must find non-investment funding sources for diversification and program development activities. The processes for seeking funds should be similar, however: (1) present investors with a description of the program; (2) identify investment dollar needs; and (3) project returns on investment.

Many sponsors of community-based centers have difficulty when attempting to define strategies for procuring and effectively using financial resources. A poorly defined or unrealistic plan for identifying reliable funding sources for both short- and long-term needs may be further complicated by inappropriate strategies for obtaining such funds.

The existence of a funding resource, such as grant funding, may encourage sponsors to engage in program planning activites. However, funding frequently is contingent upon program plans that satisfy the intent of the funding agency. When health center operations are predicated on the availability of external funding, the center may modify its own objectives to conform to funding agency objectives. As a result, the health center becomes organizationally dependent upon funding requirements that may or may not accomplish its goals or effectively serve intended patient populations. This kind of external focus is not conducive to effective internal operations, nor does it facilitate the kind of planning necessary to sustain the organization once its external funding expires.

A more viable approach, and one that addresses the long-term needs of the center, is to prepare the center's program plan and resource development strategy before applying for financial assistance. The program plan should state the center's goals and objectives as they relate to the intended service area and should outline how the center plans to achieve those objectives. Funding strategies thus are based on meeting center objectives rather than on reactions to the availability of funding—a "cart-before-the-horse" situation.

Developing an effective resource strategy entails four steps: (1) defining organizational goals and measurable time-related objectives for all programs; (2) estimating the cost associated with achieving those goals and objectives; (3) identifying potential sources of income; and (4) assessing the degree to which identified income sources are compatible with center goals and objectives.

Setting Organizational Goals and Objectives

The first step in developing an effective resource strategy is to design a plan that clearly defines organizational goals and measurable time-related objectives for all proposed programs. Each objective should be accompanied by specific activities for achieving the objective. The specification of these activities will allow the center administrator or sponsor to assess the cost involved in achieving each objective.

Estimating Cost

The second step in developing a resource strategy is to estimate the cost of achieving the goals and objectives by performing a cost analysis of the center's financial requirements. This entails developing both an operational expense budget and a capital expense budget for the entire health center. The operational budget includes all items to be expended in less than one year or with a cost of less than a preset amount (such as one hundred dollars). The capital expense budget contains all items with a useful life of more than one year and a cost above the preset amount. All costs necessary to meet the center's stated goals and objectives should be identified for purposes of the cost analysis. Operational activities should be divided categorically into multiple cost centers representing particular activities or functional units within the center. Capital requirements, which include facilities and equipment, then should be spread proportionately among cost centers. Each cost center in turn is assigned its own operational and capital expense budget.

This procedure enables administrators to estimate costs for each cost center and compare these costs with stated objectives to determine the cost-benefit of each objective and the entire program plan.

Consider the following example of applying the cost analysis approach: The health center is requested by the community to provide emergency services staffed on a 24-hour basis. The objectives of the emergency capability likely are easy to state and quantify, while the utilization objective may be more difficult to define. Assume, however, that cases the community considers to be emergencies average one to two per day (typical "emergencies" would be broken noses, heart problems, minor automobile accidents, sport injuries and farm accidents). The cost analysis shows that 24-hour coverage at the health center would cost $300,000 to $500,000 per year, or approximately $1,000 per episode. The cost analysis of an alternative to 24-hour "emergency" coverage by center staff—a physician on call for urgent cases—shows expenditures of $21,000 per year, or $40 per visit (assuming the same average number of visits). The center then must assess the financial feasibility of these two alternatives based on the community's ability (or that of insurance carriers) to pay $1,000 for emergency care capability or $40 for urgent care capability.

Once the program plan and cost analysis are complete, the center or sponsor can determine the financial resources necessary to initiate the service.

Identifying Potential Sources of Income

The third step in developing a resource strategy is to identify all potential sources of income for both development and reimbursement. Prior to 1975, the majority of dollars available to rural health were federal and state funds for public health department services. Since public health departments typically provide services to indigent populations, this funding was primarily categorical in nature and emphasized services for specific population groups (such as migrants or children) or the treatment of certain diseases and disorders (such as alcoholism and mental health) that were identified as high priority by the government funding source.

While categorical funds are still available to rural health centers, the funding thrust was altered in 1975 as evidenced by the establishment of the federal Rural Health Initiative program and the dramatic increase in private foundation sources. The new thrust, rather than providing categorical funding, financed the development of, and short-term operational deficit incurred by, a broad range of services for geographically defined service area populations.

In this chapter, developmental funding refers to funds generally used to cover program start-up costs, to purchase buildings and capital equipment and to subsidize short-term operating deficits. Short-term operating deficits generally are defined as the money needed to defray daily operating costs until the health center can generate sufficient revenue to cover those costs. The granting agency establishes a time period (usually from two to four years) it considers reasonable for subsidizing operating deficits. The following developmental funding sources are discussed: (a) federal programs; (b) state programs;

(c) foundations; (d) hospital sponsors; and (e) community sponsors. Several reimbursement sources that provide long-term operational support for the delivery of health center services also are discussed.

Developmental Resources

Federal Programs. The federal government recognized the need to improve the availability of primary care services for rural populations and began allocating funds for that purpose. The majority of federal funds for rural health care services have been distributed through the Department of Health and Human Services (DHHS) under the following programs: Rural Health Initiative (RHI), Health Underserved Rural Areas (HURA), Migrant Health Program and National Health Service Corps. The Appalachian Regional Commission (ARC) and the Community Facilities Loan Program also are supported by federal funds but are not administered by DHHS. All of the DHHS programs except HURA are currently funded. The HURA program, established in 1975 to support public and private demonstration projects and research in primary care or dental service delivery, was replaced in 1978 by the Primary Care Research and Demonstration program.

The Primary Care Research and Demonstration program supports demonstration projects involving innovative methods for providing primary health services and dental health services to medically underserved populations. It also funds research on existing or new and innovative methods of delivering these services. Only existing organizations are eligible for this support; grant funds cannot be used to cover general start-up costs for new health centers. Fifty-six projects were being funded by this program at the end of 1980.

The Rural Health Initiative program, created in 1975, provides developmental funding for rural health center sponsors. The intent of this program is to improve access to primary health care services in rural medically underserved areas and to foster community-based health care delivery systems. To date, the program has funded the development of 571 rural health centers. The Rural Health Initiative program also encourages health center sponsors to consider conjoint funding in which the applicant applies for more than one type of federal funding. For example, a health center could apply for Rural Health Initiative funds, the assignment of National Health Service Corps personnel and a facilities loan under the Community Facilities Loan Program. (The Hemmingford case study illustrates conjoint funding.)

The Community Facilities Loan Program, a capital development program, provides low-cost loans for the construction of primary care facilities. A health center must be receiving other federal funds (through RHI or the Migrant Health Program) to be eligible for a loan under this program.

Another major source of federal developmental funding is the Appalachian Regional Commission (ARC). This organization was created in 1965 to address development problems in the Appalachian region and is a partnership of 13 Appalachian state governments. In addition to rural primary care center funding, the commission funds manpower development, preventive health and emergency medical services.

Rural health centers also are eligible for federal categorical funds. Categorical funds are distributed to health centers based on the number of projected encounters with members of the defined target population or on some other basis specified in the categorical program. While categorical funds usually are provided by the federal government, program administration typically is assigned to individual state agencies.

State Programs. Several states have allocated funds for primary care development in rural areas and/or have created offices of rural health. These states include: Alabama, Arkansas, California, Colorado, Missouri, North Carolina, North Dakota and Oregon. In North Carolina, for example, the Office of Rural Health has provided developmental funds for 28 rural health sites and works with local communities in developing programs and identifying funding sources.

The implications of participating in and relying on state and federal funding are similar. Funding is contingent on the economic and political climate and therefore is subject to change. Under the Reagan Administration, for example, federal health program funding probably will be reduced. One possible option being considered for disbursing available federal funds is the block grant method under which a state distributes and administers the federal funds. Substantial changes in levels and methods of federal funding, such as the block grant approach, will pose problems for rural primary care centers relying on federal funding for development and continuing operation.

Foundations. During the 1970s, foundations became an important developmental funding resource for rural primary care. While foundations may operate under broad charters, their funding generally is limited to specific areas of interest as defined by the foundation's board of directors. In contrast to the federal government, foundations are generally more flexible in administering their programs. They are able to respond more readily to changing environmental priorities and as a rule require fewer and less detailed reports. For these reasons, foundation funding is an attractive source of support for rural health projects.

Of the more than 20,000 foundations in the United States, only a few have made substantial contributions to health care. Three foundations that have made a substantial amount of money available for rural health care programs are the W. K. Kellogg Foundation, the Robert Wood Johnson Foundation and the Kresge Foundation. The Kresge Foundation is an example of a national foundation that awards funds for construction and/or renovation of facilities and the purchase of major equipment and real estate to established organizations with a positive track record. The W. K. Kellogg Foundation, one of the five largest in the nation, supports projects in three areas: agriculture, education and health. In 1976, it funded the Innovations in Ambulatory Primary Care project, a national demonstration grant program that supported the development of 20 innovative primary care projects. The Robert Wood Johnson Foundation supports only health care projects and, with the W. K. Kellogg Foundation, has been one of the leading benefactors of health care services in underserved areas. In 1975, the Robert Wood Johnson Foundation funded the Rural Community Practice Models Program, a national demonstration grant program that supported the planning and development of 13 primary care practice organizations. Foundation grants traditionally have provided developmental support and should be considered only as a source of short-term funding.

Sponsoring Organizations: Hospitals. Hospitals have been a source of developmental funding for rural health centers and in some cases will consider long-term deficit funding. One reason hospitals may contribute to site development is to increase their referral base. The location of a primary care site in an underserved portion of the hospital's service area is a strategy to increase market share through center physician referrals of patients to the hospital.

In addition to providing direct financial support for a health center's operations, a hospital may provide services such as part- or full-time management assistance, training and continuing education for center personnel, computer access and shared service arrangements for ancillary and support services. Finally, some hospitals are affiliated with residency training programs and may provide physician resources or recruitment services for the health center. The Lutheran Hospital and Lakeview Hospital case studies illustrate financing by hospitals.

Sponsoring Organizations: Community Groups. Community residents often are actively involved in a rural health center's start-up. Community groups also can be a means to access valuable community financial resources. Community fund-raising drives not only provide a strong financial resource base but also are an excellent marketing tool for increasing health center recognition and utilization. Successful fund-raising campaigns provide evidence of strong community support, and this evidence usually is necessary for receiving grant funding. Community fund-raising drives typically raise developmental funds for facility construction, expansion or renovation, or for the acquisition of equipment. If there is strong community support, long-term operational funds may be available through local tax revenues or other sources. The Hemmingford and Cape Meares case studies illustrate two health centers that rely heavily on community fund-raising.

Reimbursement Resources

Reimbursement for services rendered may be provided on a prospective or retrospective basis, but historically has been available only retrospectively. In general, reimbursement should be considered long-term operational funding. Reimbursement resources available to health centers include (a) federal programs; (b) Blue Cross/Blue Shield; (c) private insurance groups; (d) self-insurance plans; (e) prepaid programs; and (f) payment by the service recipient (self-pay).

In general, health centers have been reimbursed under the same criteria as private physician groups delivering primary care services. This segment of the health care delivery system—primary care—has been largely overlooked by the health insurance industry since the major focus of insurance has been the more financially catastrophic illnesses that require hospitalization and specialty physician intervention. This focus has placed the burden of payment for primary care services, especially preventive and health maintenance services, on the consumer or federal programs such as Medicare and Medicaid.

Federal Programs. Federal reimbursement programs assume health insurance coverage responsibility for high-risk groups and for military employees. Medicare provides insurance coverage for those over 65 years of age, as well as for certain disabled persons, while Medicaid covers the medically indigent. Military employees are covered under the CHAMPUS program. Federal reimbursement programs typically are administered by an intermediary, such as Blue Cross/Blue Shield.

Part A of the Medicare program provides reimbursement for inpatient hospital care and hospital-related services; Part B provides reimbursement for physician services. Under Part A, a hospital receives direct reimbursement after a covered service has been provided and after the patient has paid the deductible portion of the expense. The patient is responsible for all noncovered hospital charges as well as for co-payment following hospitalization for more than 60 days. Only a health center owned and operated by a hospital is eligible for reimbursement under Part A.

Under Part B, the patient is, at minimum, responsible for an annual deductible and a 20 percent co-payment of the allowable charges. If a health center elects to accept assignment, reimbursement for those charges allowed under Medicare is sent directly to the health center, and the health center is legally obligated to write off the amount disallowed by Medicare. For example, a health center sends Medicare a $30 charge for a visit by patient x, who has already satisfied the annual deductible. Medicare's allowable charge for the particular service rendered to this patient is $20. The health center receives $16 in reimbursement and can bill the patient for 20 percent of the allowable charge, or $4. The disallowed $10 must be written off by the health center as a contractual allowance. If a center does not elect assignment, the patient is responsible for the full charge for the service rendered. Having satisfied the annual deductible, the patient receives a check directly from Medicare for 80 percent of the allowable charge ($16 in the example above).

Because the Medicaid program is funded and administered jointly by the states and the federal government, eligibility and coverage vary by state. A center elects whether to participate in the Medicaid program. For a participating center, Medicaid provides a reimbursement rate as payment in full for the covered services; the rate is usually less than the health center's actual charge. If a center does not participate, patients cannot use Medicaid to pay for services rendered. In any event, if Medicaid reimbursement does not cover actual costs, the center must decide if other patient groups should subsidize Medicaid patients.

There are several disadvantages to participating in the Medicare and Medicaid programs. For example, centers generally require additional staff for related bookkeeping functions. There is also a time lapse between the delivery of a service and reimbursement for that service by Medicare and Medicaid. These reimbursement programs also are subject to funding cuts and delays, rendering the reimbursement schedule unpredictable.

Hospital-owned centers may have a reimbursement advantage over centers sponsored by hospitals or other organizations. If a hospital-owned center is considered to be an outpatient department, the center may qualify for higher reimbursement rates. This may be due to cost-based reimbursement and the way in which hospitals allocate their costs to maximize reimbursement. The University Medical Center case study illustrates this difference.

Private Insurance. Private insurance companies provide insurance packages to experience-rated and pooled-risk groups for which the actual claims experience is less than premium revenue. Experience rating typically is used for large employer groups and premiums are based on the actual cost experience of the group. Premiums for small employer groups (typically organizations with 50 to 100 employees) are determined by the pool in which they are placed by the insurance company. For example, a retailer employing 50 people would be assigned to a pool of retailers of approximately the same size, and the premium would be based on the experience of the entire pool. Insurance companies minimize risk to themselves by carefully tailoring their packages to the risks inherent in different employee groups and/or by providing reimbursement at a fixed dollar amount (or indemnity) so that the insured is responsible for costs above that amount. Health insurance policies vary in coverage of non-hospital services and in co-insurance and deductible features. One problem for health centers is that patients may not understand the kinds of services covered and the policy's dollar limitations and are reluctant to assume responsibility for paying noncovered charges.

Blue Cross/Blue Shield. Blue Cross/Blue Shield is a private, nonprofit health insurer comprised of individual plans incorporated at the state level. Blue Cross covers hospital services while Blue Shield covers physician services. Health center services typically are covered under Blue Shield, with coverage ranging from minimal to comprehensive. Although coverage depends on the policy, most plans have emphasized inpatient hospital and specialty care coverage and minimized coverage for ambulatory primary care services. Although Blue Cross uses an experience rating method, premiums are based primarily on a community rating or the pooled experience of all groups within a particular region. Participating health centers receive direct reimbursement at rates established by the local Blue Cross/Blue Shield plan. In the case of non-participating health centers, Blue Cross/Blue Shield reimburses the patient, who is directly responsible for all health center charges. Because of variations in Blue Cross/Blue Shield plans and uninformed patients, determination of coverage is difficult for the health center and additional staff is required to ascertain coverage and complete insurance forms.

Self-Insured Plans. Major nonunion employers are becoming increasingly interested in self-insured plans. Corporations are concerned about the high cost of providing health insurance to their employees and recognize that preventive health care, typically not covered under commercial insurance policies, influences employee health status and productivity.

The advent of self-insurance plans represents one response to the high cost of health insurance. These plans specify the kinds of services (provided to the insured employees) that are reimbursable. Funds are set aside by the corporation for paying claims. The corporation usually contracts with an insurance agency to manage the administrative aspects of the plan. Under this type of arrangement, the health center bills the corporation's insurance plan directly for reimbursement for covered services. Health centers serving large numbers of participating corporate employees may be able to influence program coverage and reimbursement levels if the corporation specifies, at a local level, which services are reimbursable.

Prepaid Plans. A center may contract with a local group of people to provide a set of services on a prepaid basis. Relationships with health maintenance organizations are an example. While the number of health maintenance organizations is increasing rapidly, they tend to capture a small share of the total market (some metropolitan areas, such as Minneapolis/St. Paul, are an exception). Medicare and Medicaid also have entered into prepaid contracts on a demonstration basis. By receiving a predetermined monthly fee per enrollee, the health center assumes the risk that fees will cover the cost of providing services to these enrollees.

Health centers can benefit from prepaid plans in several ways. First, centers experience a positive cash flow since payment is received prior to the delivery of service. Second, centers can accrue additional interest through earlier investment and can devote fewer resources to collection activities. And third, centers can predict and budget revenues more accurately than they can under retrospective reimbursement arrangements. Cost-effectiveness also can be promoted through prepaid arrangements if centers encourage enrollees to use lower-cost preventive services rather than more costly inpatient services.

Direct Payment by Patients (Self-Pay). Self-pay patients are directly responsible for reimbursing the center for services received. In addition, patients with insurance coverage must pay out-of-pocket for services not covered by their insurance plan. In either case, a center should establish and publish guidelines for billing frequency and for the collection of problem accounts. To avoid high collection and credit costs, many health centers require payment at the time of service. Extension of credit implies that center resources must be allocated to billing. Most health centers receive up to 50 percent of all service revenues from self-pay patients.

Identifying a Compatible Resource Base

Upon completion of the cost analysis and the identification of potential funding and reimbursement sources, the fourth and final step for the center is to identify a resource base through which the center can accomplish its objectives. This resource base consists of short-term (one to three years) and long-term (three to 25 years) sources of income, including reimbursement revenues that can be used for both capital and operating expenses.

Developmental Resources

There are five major considerations in establishing a compatible resource base that will optimize the relationship between financing and operations:

☐ The degree of consistency between center objectives and those of the funding agencies

☐ The probability of the funding being long-term

☐ The image of the center

☐ The funding cycle and operational restrictions or policies of each funding source

☐ The ability to achieve financial self-sufficiency.

Consistency Between Center and Agency Objectives. The first task in identifying a compatible resource base is to evaluate the center's objectives compared with those of the funding agency. Consistency of objectives is essential to developing a positive relationship between the funding agency and the applicant. Many rural health centers have solicited resources on the basis of ill-defined and/or humanistically articulated objectives. Upon receipt of a financial award, the center may discover that the funding contract contains objectives and reporting requirements that conflict with the center's intent and resources. To avoid this conflict, centers must clearly specify their objectives and compare those objectives to funding program criteria. Rejecting funding sources that are inappropriate for accomplishing health center objectives will save time, energy and money.

Assessing the Probability of Long-Term Funding. The second task is to determine whether the granting agency is providing short- or long-term financial support. Health centers must ensure the existence of both short- and long-term funding resources to cover anticipated expenses before they begin operations. Reimbursement programs such as Medicare, Medicaid, Blue Cross/Blue Shield and private insurance carriers are a more reliable source for long-term funding than are demonstration grant programs through private foundations, which are best viewed as sources for short-term support. Program goals requiring long-term support may be incompatible with short-term funding resources.

Consider the following illustration: A health center identifies and obtains sufficient short-term developmental funding to finance facility construction, equipment and initial operating deficits but fails to identify and obtain the long-term funding required to offset the economics of its service area population, which can barely support the salary for one physician let alone support the staff and overhead for a center. In this case, the center may be forced to close after the short-term funding has expired. Conversely, a lack of short-term start-up funding for initial capital and operating expenses often prevents health care centers from being established despite the existence of reasonable long-term funding bases.

Careful consideration should be given to identifying both short- and long-term funding sources and matching these sources with health center needs and objectives. Failure to do so may force centers to discontinue certain services after their grants expire. (The Cape Meares and Lutheran Hospital case studies illustrate this problem.)

Determining the Appropriate Image. The third task in identifying a compatible resource base is to determine whether the funding source is compatible with the health center image, which in turn depends on the expectations of the service population. This step requires that the health center (1) determine the image desired or necessary to enhance community acceptance and utilization and (2) evaluate potential funding sources in terms of their likely effect on that image. Certain funding sources carry negative connotations among residents of small and/or rural communities. These sources may be perceived as "government," "free-care," "needy," "welfare," "volunteer," "research" or "university." Centers relying on funding sources that engender negative connotations among the community will have a difficult time gaining community support. Certain segments of the community may not use a health center because of negative perceptions. A center with a multifaceted resource base is most likely to develop an image that is compatible with a broad range of community perceptions and expectations. On the other hand, a center using a single source of grant income as its primary funding resource will most likely develop a stereotypic community image, which may or may not be consistent with the organization's objectives and may influence program or market expansion efforts. (The Cape Meares and Lutheran Hospital case studies illustrate problems associated with community perceptions.)

Assessing the Policies of Each Funding Source. The fourth task in identifying a compatible resource base is to assess the policies of each potential funding agency and how they relate to the objectives and resources of the health center. This is important since the funding cycles and reporting requirements may necessitate certain changes in a health center's planning and/or operational procedures. Many grant programs are funded on an annual basis or only at the start of a particular grant cycle. To be eligible for these programs, a center must develop plans, objectives, budgets and evaluation activities that conform to the funding cycle of the granting agency. For many centers, this requires substantial planning as well as possible organizational changes, including fiscal year alterations, multiple program budgets and often multiple audits.

The policies of a grant agency may require that applications be submitted before the start of a funding cycle and that the grant-related program be operational shortly after acceptance of the award. In fact, some grantees have received grant award notices for programs that were to be operational before any financial remuneration was available. This creates a dilemma: either fail to meet the award conditions or borrow money to finance initial cash requirements, although the interest payments on the loan may be a disallowed expense under the grant. Organizations that apply for such grants face these and similiar difficulties unless other portions of the resource base can be used to cover the nonreimbursable expenses generated in meeting the grant criteria.

The most notable examples of dissonant funding conditions occur in government grant programs that are categorical in nature. The development or expansion of services for a specific population group (such as the poor, the elderly or rural communities) often is a direct response to the current political climate regarding categorical funding priorities. Health centers may develop substantial programs to address the needs of these populations without considering the potential long-term viability of either the program or the health center itself should the funding no longer be available. Because such funding usually is directed at a population that has difficulty paying for health care services, the funding agency offers few incentives to make the program self-sufficient from reimbursement sources. In some governmental grant programs, a disincentive for financial self-sufficiency actually exists since the premise for funding is the inability of the targeted population or local sources to pay for the care delivered. When new government officials are elected, it is likely that the categorical program will be discontinued or that its objectives and funding practices will be substantially altered. The center's viability may be jeopardized when single or multiple programs are discontinued or their funding terminated.

Federal grant programs often are designed to provide health care services to medically underserved areas. This implies that the potential for health center funding will be directly related to the center's ability to demonstrate a real need for the services. In fact, health centers (or sponsors) located in areas with the greatest demonstrated need are encouraged to apply over health centers in areas with less demonstrated need. Unfortunately, areas with the greatest need for medical care systems are also areas with a limited range of available supportive services and a severely limited capability for developing a viable health care delivery organization. As a result, successful applicants from underserved areas often face a dilemma of having adequate financial resources but a shortage of other resources for an effective health care delivery system. Many health center sponsors in underserved and medically unsophisticated communities set goals that are inconsistent with the resources available in the area for achieving those goals. This creates an imbalance between a grantor's expectations and the grantee's capabilities and hinders the development of an adequate health care delivery system. It is important that the health center's resource base be developed with a clear perspective of the center's ability to convert funding resources into well-trained personnel and, subsequently, into effective, efficient services.

Federal agencies that award grants on the basis of demonstrated need often evaluate the health center on the basis of service delivery to the target population. The assumption of the grant agency usually is that services delivered will reduce the need upon which the grant award was based. However, the services that are initiated or expanded with the funding may not always be in the best interest of the health center or the community. For example, the services provided may not actually reduce the need demonstrated in the community; or the health center may not be able to convert the services into reimbursement that will support its future funding base. A grant awarded on the basis of need but evaluated on the basis of service delivery therefore can lead to conflict within the health center and within the community. (The Montgomery County Hospital case study illustrates this situation.)

It is important for a health center to be aware of a potential funding source's basis for awarding the grant and its criteria for evaluating the use of those funds. The grant agency's criteria should be compatible with the health center's objectives and long-term funding base before the source receives serious consideration. An applicant organization that can evaluate performance by both service and reimbursement objectives is most likely to be an organization whose expectations are compatible with those of the granting agency.

Achieving Financial Self-Sufficiency. The final task in developing a compatible resource base is to actively pursue a course leading to planned financial self-sufficiency. While financial self-sufficiency depends upon generating revenues to cover the costs of service provision, grant agencies (and health centers) may use differing criteria to evaluate the achievement of self-sufficiency. For example, financial self-sufficiency is defined by the Department of Health and Human Services as the extent to which billings equal charges. However, not all federal programs use the same definition. The Appalachian Regional Commission states that self-sufficiency is achieved when a center is no longer dependent on short-term grant support, although funding under long-term programs (such as the Rural Health Initiative program) is acceptable under its definition. The Rural Health Initiative program has determined that centers will continue to be eligible for funding as long as the practices are "efficient." Efficiency is interpreted to mean that, after two years of full operation, no more than 20 percent of the health center's total ambulatory care costs are allocated for administrative expenses. Health centers also have varying definitions of self-sufficiency. (For example, the Brushwood Health Station sponsor defines self-sufficiency as the integration of the center's operational costs into the public health department's budget.)

Generally, government and foundation grants awarded for center start-up purposes will subsidize a center's short-term operational deficits until its operations can be supported by program-generated reimbursement. Difficulties arise when the self-sufficiency objective is not clearly defined by either party or when attempts are made to alter the agreed upon definition of self-sufficiency.

Problems arise when grant agencies alter their original funding criteria and in doing so actually encourage programs or services that cannot be sustained without subsidization. The health center then will be dependent on the funding agency for the survival and direction of these programs. The greater the number of services dependent on subsidized funding, the greater the dependence of the health center on the funding agency. This fiscal dependency reduces the subsidized center's (or sponsor's) ability to develop independent judgment, self-direction and earned success. The center becomes, in essence, a governmental service program administered by a community organization. The inability of the center to develop its own objectives fosters a conflict between the short-term need for maintaining a financial base (by adopting the objectives of the funding agency) and the long-range need for developing an independently viable resource plan that could sustain the center should grant funds be reduced or discontinued.

The dependency issue also arises in other funding relationships, such as when a large organization like a hospital supports a smaller ambulatory care organization. The hospital often enters into the relationship because the needs of the two organizations seem to be compatible. The hospital may become disenchanted when the sponsored ambulatory care organization drains hospital resources because of high overhead costs and low productivity. The hospital's ability to balance internal versus external expenditures may reach a critical point when the hospital's medical staff and/or its departments request resources that are unavailable for internal use because they are being used by the external facility. The resulting conflict usually is resolved either by severing the funding arrangements or by assimilating the health center into the hospital.

A viable health center must maintain goals and objectives that are consistent with the broad-based purpose of an ambulatory primary care center. When a center becomes dependent upon the objectives of an external funding source or a larger organization, it will likely respond to the needs of the sponsoring organization rather than to the community's needs or its own long-term need for viability. In such cases, the center's resource base becomes its reason for existence. The University Medical Center, Montgomery County Hospital and Lutheran Hospital case studies illustrate some aspects of this problem.

Two requirements most often overlooked when evaluating grant resources are the personnel and the management skills needed to fulfill the administrative conditions of a grant. Both the sponsoring organization and the primary care center should estimate the skills, information systems and management control mechanisms needed to track the programmatic objectives established in the initial plan. They must then carefully evaluate the extra requirements of the grant agency and how the requirements may tax those skills and systems. Grant recipients may find themselves in financial difficulty when the award budget fails to meet the increased costs of information retrieval or when attendant accounting, statistical reporting and regulatory administration activities are incompatible with the size and resources of the recipient organization. A growing organization, as measured by an increase in the number of patients served, the services offered and the financial data requested by the granting agency, may face a problem of diminishing returns as financial support from the grant decreases while the level of expertise required for and the expense of reporting to the grant organization increase.

The common thread in these five considerations for a developmental resource base is the potential incompatibility of a grantee's organizational objectives or operational policies with those of the grantor. The success of any funding relationship will depend on the ability of each organization to respond effectively to the requirements of the other and the ability of each to clearly identify its intent and direction as it relates to the intent and direction of the other organization.

Reimbursement Resources

Given the prevalence of fee-for-service financing mechanisms and the evolution of third-party carriers as primary reimbursement agents, health care organizations must develop strategies for maximizing third-party reimbursement. A hospital's chief financial officer often is evaluated on his or her ability to maximize reimbursement by developing an expense reporting strategy that provides the hospital with an improved reimbursement-to-cost ratio. A similar situation exists in the provision of ambulatory care services. However, the rules governing this area differ somewhat, and the sophistication of the players is more likely to be in health care delivery or management than in financing.

A substantial portion of a hospital's revenue is generated by payments from insurers such as Blue Cross, commercial companies and federal programs such as Medicare and Medicaid. These insurers provide reimbursement for a wide range of services for hospitalized patients. Ambulatory primary care services, however, are seldom covered, especially preventive care, health maintenance, routine examinations, counseling or health screening. The resulting financial impact on the ambulatory primary care center is a potpourri that may include partial reimbursement, co-payments, deductibles or no payment provisions for ambulatory primary care services in the patient's insurance coverage. To complicate the matter, most small rural health centers, because of budgetary limitations, cannot support a highly trained full-time financial manager. Consequently, the majority of health centers must rely on individuals with limited financial management experience to determine the reimbursement mix of the patient population and develop a strategy for maximizing the center's reimbursement level.

Developing a reimbursement strategy for an ambulatory primary care center begins with a detailed listing of the services to be provided, the probable sources of reimbursement for the services and an estimate of patient demand for those services. A successful strategy depends on the ability of the organization to match services rendered with the ability and willingness of reimbursers to pay for those services. In general, health centers should not develop a service unless reimbursement sources are available in sufficient quantity to support that service when the organization's capacity to provide it or the projected demand for it has been reached. Ideally, once capacity and demand have been reached, the fees established for services should produce a total net income equal to or exceeding the total net expense for delivering those services at capacity.

The cost of delivering services should be adjusted to maximize third-party reimbursement when reimbursement is available for a covered service. For example, if it costs a health center $9 to perform a specific laboratory test while third-party payers have set a $10 reimbursement rate for this test, the health center should set its charge to maximize this reimbursement. If delivered services are not covered by third-party payers or if reimbursement levels vary among payers, fees should be set at a level comparable to other providers in the area.

Health center administrators must be careful to set adequate fee levels to help ensure continuing financial viability. Third-party payers often use "usual, customary and reasonable" charges in setting future reimbursement levels. If a health center's current fees are set at levels below or just at cost, the increasing cost of delivering services will soon exceed reimbursement for those services. The Hemmingford case study illustrates this problem.

Once the expense of delivering services has been determined, fees should be set at a level that will, at minimum, cover those costs. This approach assumes that a health center will be able to recover 100 percent of its costs by charging at 100 percent of costs. Since collection efforts rarely achieve a 100-percent level, the health center must consider how it can best maximize reimbursement from all sources to cover its costs.

In summary, a reimbursement strategy designed to maximize total fee-for-service reimbursement from all sources must consider three factors:

☐ The mix of payers for the potential patient population

☐ The kinds of services each payer covers

☐ The usual and customary fees for specific services charged by other providers in the area.

A financing approach that is more predictable than maximizing fee-for-service reimbursement is to recover the cost of the service on a predetermined charge basis from the organization or individual requesting the service. This approach can be used when the service provider and the insuring entity are operating in a coordinated fashion. One example is the health maintenance organization (HMO) that offers a guaranteed set of inpatient and ambulatory care services for a predetermined, prepaid fee. Substantial financial advantages accrue to the developing health center that contracts with an HMO since payment schedules are predictable and since costs can be related to charges. The health center can determine in advance the cost of a particular set of services and then can negotiate a predetermined monthly payment for each HMO patient enrolled at the center. As an alternative approach, a center may choose to participate with an independent practice association HMO, which allows the center to charge a predetermined fee for each service rendered on a fee-for-service basis.

Both of these mechanisms—the predetermined prepaid fee and the predetermined fee-for-service charge—enable the health center to develop a consistent reimbursement structure based on operating costs rather than determining charges on the basis of who pays the bill. Rural health center sponsors should carefully evaluate HMO options for financing. Most rural areas lack the insurance and/or population bases necessary to support an HMO and few centers can provide a sufficient scope of services to qualify for capitation contracts with third-party payers. Prepaid arrangements often are complex and risky. The organizational mechanisms needed to reduce financial risk (such as utilization controls) are difficult to implement and maintain. However, prepayment can offer positive financial incentives to participate if a center can expand into new market areas once it is established and if the prepaid system is carefully planned, monitored and controlled. Health centers wishing to explore prepaid options should seek experienced, professional assistance.

The long-term viability of a health center is directly related to its ability to recover costs in a consistent manner. The ability of an organization to establish charges on the basis of an awareness of costs rather than on market conditions constitutes the most effective strategy for long-term financial success.

Expanding the Resource Base

Once a health center has developed a short-term resource base to support its initial development and operations and is fully operational, the ensuing period of patient and revenue growth (years one to three), if efficiently managed, should move the resource base from short-term grant funding to long-term reimbursement funding. Given the socio-economic status and size of the population base, some rural areas may never be able to support center services without subsidization. However, sponsors and center administrators should make every effort to explore options that will reduce the center's reliance on grant subsidies.

An organization is considered to be financially viable at the existing level of operation once the income from reimbursement sources (insurance, patients or prepaid contractual services) equals its operating expenses. Many administrators assume that, once that point is reached, the operation is successful and an effective management strategy consists of maintaining the status quo by increasing charges and, consequently, revenue to cover increases in expenses. Yet this strategy is inconsistent with public and private efforts to contain health care costs, which have exceeded cost escalations in other sectors of the economy and continue to consume an increasing share of the gross national product.

The status quo assumption also does not account for other variables, such as market competition or reductions in payments from federal and private third-party insurance carriers, that may affect a center's financial viability. Outcomes related to these variables may include: (1) a slower increase in charges than in costs; (2) a decrease in coverage for certain services or populations; and/or (3) a temporary decrease in payment for all services. A health center must constantly measure its impact on the existing market and must continually develop and expand its resource base if it is to achieve, maintain and strengthen its viability in the face of a changing environment. It is not enough for a health center to be financially self-sufficient at the existing level of operations; future self-sufficiency will depend on its ability to anticipate changing environmental demands and adapt to these demands before they reach critical levels.

Health centers can facilitate the development of an expanded resource base by adhering to four principles:

☐ Increase profit margins by increasing efficiency per unit of service without unnecessarily increasing charges.

☐ Reduce the expense per service by spreading fixed costs over a greater number of services.

☐ Directly increase revenue by adding new services that require less expense than the income generated.

☐ Maximize the growth produced from retained earnings by effective profit management.

The first principle requires an evaluation of the efficiency with which current services are delivered. Some areas to be examined for possible improvements in efficiency are the roles and scheduling of personnel and the patient flow. For example, the delivery of preventive care and assessment services by nurses and mid-level practitioners rather than by physicians results in a much lower per-unit cost. Another efficiency improvement area might be a center's hours of operations, which could be changed to conform with peak load utilization. The nurse practitioner in the Tehama County case study realizes that, because patients were unlikely to keep appointments at the health station during the hottest time of the day, it is more efficient for the center to be open early in the morning and late in the evening.

The second principle assumes that there are certain costs that will not increase when the volume of service increases. These costs are generally termed fixed costs and include rent or mortgage payments, utilities, equipment and administration. A center that increases patient volume by 20 percent may only increase such variable costs as personnel and supplies. The 20 percent increase in revenue is then offset by a less than 20 percent increase in costs, which generates a greater proportion of revenue-to-expense through a lower fixed cost per patient visit. If, however, the increase in patient volume necessitates a proportional increase in personnel, supplies, space, equipment and administration, there is no economic advantage to the increase in patient volume. If a wide range of ambulatory care services (such as nutrition, counseling, dental, health education, physical therapy services) can be offered at the center without increasing fixed costs, the fixed costs attributable to each service or cost center will be lower. In addition, a wide range of services may offer opportunities for instituting profit centers through industrial health programs, school system health supports, health maintenance organizations and other prepaid contracts.

The third principle entails a decision to add new services, which should be carefully evaluated by the administrator to ensure that these services actually generate greater income than required expenses. Health centers tend to underestimate the costs of initiating new ventures by failing to anticipate all consequences flowing from these ventures. All possible short- and long-term costs and revenue sources must be considered before a new program is undertaken. For example, a dental service unit generally entails less expense than income generated once the initial equipment costs have been absorbed. Health centers must consider not only the need and demand for a service but also expected reimbursement sources. If, for example, the trend of third-party payers is to reimburse for dental services, it may be advantageous for the center to offer such services.

The fourth principle is based on the assumption that the health center generates more income than expense or that the health center receives payment before delivery of the service as in the case of a prepaid capitation payment from a health maintenance organization. Investing profits or cash holdings on a short- or long-term basis is essential to maximizing revenue sources. Such investments are not precluded by a nonprofit tax status so long as they are consistent with sound business judgment and support the goals of the organization. Income-generating reserve funds for capital development are a wise strategy for a growing health center that cannot look to the investor marketplace for expansion financing.

The prevalance of the fee-for-service system, where reimbursement occurs after service delivery, has encouraged the development of specialized and often isolated physician services that focus on diagnosis and treatment of particular organ systems or diseases rather than health maintenance efforts. Such fragmented responses to illness patterns in the population often create a patchwork approach to developing new services and a tenuous ability to sustain these services over the long term. A more effective approach is to anticipate and plan for a range of services that will effectively respond to the broad spectrum of health problems at the primary care level and prepare for those changes that will be required by a new health care environment.

Summary

A health center seeking to begin programs and/or diversify must carefully consider short- and long-term funding needs and resources. Careful attention to program planning (addressed in greater detail in the chapter *Managing the Future through Planned Organizational Change*) and evaluation of potential financing sources can help ensure that the financing is compatible with organizational goals and objectives, thereby enhancing the likelihood of a solid foundation and future for the health center services.

Whether a health center seeks public or private developmental financing, among the important factors to evaluate are goal and image compatability, operational restrictions and dependency on the funding sources. Reimbursement for ambulatory primary care services consists of an array of complex and confusing programs. A successful strategy for reimbursement to offset the cost of health center operations depends on the ability of the manager to match the services of the health center with the willingness of reimbursers to pay for those services.

5
Managing the Future Through Planned Organizational Change

Stephen F. Loebs, Ph.D.
Judith L. Johnson, M.A.
Rosemary L. Summers, M.P.H.

Dr. Loebs is associate professor and director of the Graduate Program in Hospital and Health Services Administration at Ohio State University, Columbus.

Ms. Johnson is a doctoral candidate in rural sociology at Ohio State University, Columbus.

Ms. Summers, formerly casebook coordinator for the Innovations in Ambulatory Primary Care project, the Hospital Research and Educational Trust, Chicago, is continuing education specialist in the Division of Community Health Service at the University of North Carolina, Chapel Hill.

Managing the Future Through Planned Organizational Change

Long-range viability—also known as staying in business over the long run—is a goal for most organizations. Unless they define goals and strategies for achieving long-range viability, organizations are almost certain to be short-timers. There is no guarantee, however, that goal and strategy definition will assure viability. The goals identified by the organization may be inappropriate and the strategies ill-conceived.

The factors necessary to keep an organization in business over a long period of time vary by type and size of organization, geographic location and characteristics of the work force. These variations complicate the task of attaining and maintaining long-range viability and make it difficult to devise neat prescriptions for success that fit every situation and organization. Rural primary health care centers are no exception. The long-range viability of these centers—their ability to continue providing health care services to defined communities over an indefinite period of time—must be an ongoing concern of both sponsors and center managers if survival, continued operations and growth are desired.

This chapter addresses three major factors that influence long-range viability: program planning, organizational growth and development and strategic planning. Through program planning, a health center makes choices even before it opens that will affect its existence and survival. Careful program planning can help a health center manager or sponsor avoid wasting resources in crisis intervention and in solving problems that need not have occurred. As does any organization, a health center moves through cycles of growth and development. The ability to respond to the needs and problems that typically arise at each cycle will in large part determine the long-range viability of the center. This chapter presents a life-cycle model of organizational growth and development typical in the rural health center setting, along with a discussion of the problems and needs unique to each stage of the cycle and the management skills needed to enable the organization to adapt to each stage. Even with careful program planning, the organization must have a mechanism to adapt to changing environmental conditions and operational experience. The strategic planning process is one mechanism by which the organization can adapt, thereby controlling its own future.

Program Planning

Program plans guide the development of the center by defining its goals and identifying the process of developing, mobilizing and utilizing resources to meet those goals. The success or failure of the program planning process therefore affects the long-range viability of rural health centers. For example, failure to carefully consider the characteristics of the service area population can produce an inappropriate provider mix and/or low center utilization and subsequent financial problems. As an illustration, the services of a full-time pediatrician in an area with a low proportion of persons under age 14 likely will be underutilized and will need to be subsidized by other health center operations.

Ideally, if time and resources permit, the program planning process would be designed and carried out by a staff member assigned that responsibility full-time. It is more likely, however, that the process will be carried out on a more informal basis as part of the total responsibility of the center administrator. Regardless of who has primary responsibility for the process, it is important to involve all persons who will make decisions on the health center's direction and operation.

While several definitions of planning have been proposed, Hyman (1976) has organized them into several models with a central theme:

☐ The process of planning is central to goal definition

☐ Planning generates alternative choices (means or strategies) to achieve an objective (goal)

☐ Planning attempts to connect existing data with needs, criteria for success, economic and political feasibility and efficient use of resources

☐ Planning stresses the future, with boundaries being defined by the planners and decision makers.

A series of steps can be used to translate the planning concept into a process. The planning process should become an ongoing, continuous management activity. As an ongoing activity, the planning process helps the organization make the essential choices that determine its courses of action, which in turn will determine its success or failure in achieving long-range viability. The program planning process consists of the following broad steps:

☐ Identify the desired status and goals. (Examples might be to improve the health status in a target population group, to increase the use of certain health care services and to continue the existence of the organization.)

☐ Determine and forecast conditions likely to occur if no action is taken.

☐ Identify resources, such as physicians, nurse practitioners, space and money, that will be necessary to achieve the stated goals.

☐ Develop alternative methods for obtaining and using these resources.

☐ Evaluate the alternatives and select the one (or a sequence) most likely to achieve the identified goals.

☐ Commence operations based upon the planning decisions.

☐ Evaluate the decisions in terms of their impact on goal achievement, and make adjustments in strategies if goals are not achieved.

Each of these broad steps contains specific tasks that, when completed, yield a fully developed program plan.* While different methods are used to accomplish these tasks, and different settings suggest different approaches, rural primary care centers should pay particular attention to four issues within the planning process as they strive for long-range viability. They are: (a) assessing the environment, (b) planning the facility, (c) developing clear goals and objectives and (d) evaluating center operations.

Assessing the Environment

Program planning directed toward achieving long-range viability should include an assessment of the environment in which the rural health center will exist. Data gathered at a national level indicate that the following socioeconomic and medical need factors exist in the rural environment:

---

*Communities or individuals engaged in planning for a rural health center can obtain detailed guidelines from *Planning and Managing Rural Health Centers* by T.L. Wade and E.F. Brooks (Ballinger Publishing Co., 1979).

Socioeconomic Factors:

☐ The rural population accounts for 40 percent of all Americans living below the poverty level.

☐ Minority groups and the elderly comprise relatively greater numbers of the rural poor than they do the urban poor.

☐ Low income levels, dispersed populations and lack of transportation severely limit access to needed services of all kinds.

Medical Need Factors:

☐ All U.S. counties with infant mortality rates that are double the national average are rural counties.

☐ Rural residents have higher rates of chronic disease, morbidity and mortality due to accidents.

☐ Health resources have steadily declined in rural areas as indicated by a declining physician-to-population ratio. (Lichty and Zuvekas, 1980)

The environment in which the rural health center characteristically must operate and achieve viability makes it crucial for the health center to carefully assess its local environment. The center should first define the geographic and population boundaries to be served. This definition will help determine the mix of services needed, demand projections for those services, staffing plans, needed financial resources and the kind of physical facility required. After the service area has been defined, the local socioeconomic and medical need factors should be identified.

It is also important to examine local socio-political factors for their possible effects on the center. Conflicts among vested interest groups may affect center utilization if these groups are defined as part of the target population. One study showed that limiting services to certain income and racial groups caused disagreements as to who should be receiving services (Gurwitz and Dennis, 1975). Conflict between service recipients and nonrecipients limited community involvement, fostered hostility toward the center and eventually caused financial problems.

Planning the Facility

One of the first issues faced in planning for community-based health services is a facility. Many communities believe that attractive medical facilities are the only important ingredient in recruiting a physician. For this reason, they often build or remodel a facility before program planning is initiated. The facility may be planned with the solo practitioner in mind rather than as a fully developed, comprehensive health center. This often results in a facility that is too small for multiple providers and ancillary service development. Conversely, some communities that build large, new facilities find it difficult to support their high overhead costs in the face of slowly growing patient revenues.

While any facility is tangible evidence of progress, several program planning decisions should be made before a facility is established. However, because many of the planning steps necessary for a successful operation are not as tangible as facility procurement, it often is difficult to focus those involved in planning (and particularly the community leadership) on other program planning decisions. These decisions include projected number of providers, services to be offered, projected utilization and proximity to the major service area population. Unless facility development is based on these decisions, a community may find itself with a facility with limited growth potential or one too large to support financially.

Developing Clear Goals and Objectives

Once health center planners have defined those factors influencing the delivery of health services, they must specify the goals of the organization. These goals should be consistent with both the needs and resource limitations identified during the environmental assessment. Next, objectives leading to the achievement of each goal should be formulated. Objectives should be specific, measurable and time-phased. Each objective therefore should include a statement of what will be done, how it will be measured and when it will be accomplished. Third, the specific activities or tasks necessary for accomplishing the objective should be identified.

The leap from assessing factors likely to influence the delivery of services to specifying goals, objectives and activities can be the most difficult part of the planning process. Persons participating in the planning process often disagree over the best way to meet the community's health care needs. Rarely is this conflict addressed during the planning process, however. Such disagreements must be addressed and resolved during the planning stage, since they can result in limited community support for the center and even sabotage center programs. Success of the health center will depend on the planner's ability to identify these conflicts and negotiate their resolution at the outset.

Once center goals, objectives and activities have been specified and agreed upon, strategies for implementing the activities must be developed. Strategies for implementation—including financing, personnel recruitment and retention and organizational design—are discussed in other chapters of this book.

Evaluating Operations

The planning process must include a mechanism or method for measuring goal and objective attainment so that new plans or program modifications can be undertaken. The evaluation can be elaborate or abbreviated depending on available time and resources. When establishing an evaluation plan, health center managers or sponsors should be fully aware of the kinds and amounts of data that will be needed for the evaluation and the resources needed to obtain the data. An evaluation plan that calls for the analysis of treated diseases must also provide for the collection of the data. In general, the smaller the health center, the more limited will be its administrative and support services, implying a simple evaluation plan with minimal data requirements.

Deniston and Rosenstock (1978) indicate that a program should be evaluated with respect to objectives (that is, outputs, outcomes, goals) and in terms of the appropriateness, adequacy, effectiveness and efficiency of the objectives. Program *appropriateness* must be evaluated in two separate contexts. In the first, the desirability of the program or objective is assessed in an absolute sense. For example, is it desirable for a health center to offer emergency services regardless of the cost of providing those services? In the second context, the desirability of the program or objective is evaluated relative to other programs or objectives. For example, if the cost of providing emergency services exceeds their generated revenue, is it desirable to continue these services through subsidies from other revenue-producing services?

Adequacy is the measure of the extent to which the program is directed toward meeting the objectives. *Effectiveness* measures the extent to which objectives are actually attained. The *efficiency* of a program reflects the relationship between inputs and outcomes. Efficiency is the relationship between resources expended and net attainment of program objectives and represents an average cost with respect to the program or objective being measured.

While this approach is complex and somewhat abstract, it does yield a comprehensive evaluation of all health center objectives. Other approaches, such as obtaining trend line information on health status indicators among the target population, on utilization of services and on client satisfaction, may be less expensive and adequately serve a health center's evaluation needs.

As in other enterprises, the evaluation of organizational success and viability also must include financial self-sufficiency and, more longitudinally, long-range financial viability. The mission of rural primary care health centers includes more than financial self-sufficiency, however. They are established primarily to provide a needed service. Evaluation therefore must determine if needed services are used by those who need them, and if not, why. This information is used by sponsors and management to alter the services provided or the methods by which they are provided. This illustrates the circular or iterative dimension of program planning—the process is never complete because new information is constantly being received that may require changes in the total program. Organizations that recognize this dimension are most likely to be viable and responsive to their constituencies over the long term.

Organizational Change and Growth

The factors and decisions that affect long-range viability depend in part on the ability of health centers to adapt to change and growth. For example, a health center will need to adjust its operations in response to changes in the type and needs of its clients, to changes in funding sources and requirements and to changes in utilization patterns. If a center cannot successfully adapt to new demands and adopt new strategies for survival and growth, viability may be beyond its reach. The stability of a center depends greatly on the willingness of its staff to be involved in and support new ventures, policy changes and work procedures.

The Process of Organizational Change

Organizational change is a continuous process of adapting work procedures, programs, staffing assignments, external relationships and behavior patterns in response to factors in the organization's environment. This environment may include funding sources, other health care organizations that provide needed services, providers contracting with the center and clients. Aiken and Hage (1971) and Hage (1980) identify four stages in the process of organizational change: evaluation, initiation, implementation and routinization.

Evaluation

During the evaluation stage, the organization becomes aware that a problem exists. This awareness stems from a perceived gap between expected and actual performance in achieving stated program objectives. Whether the gap is identified by the formal evaluation methods described previously or through informal information sources, current and projected performance must be evaluated if appropriate and required organizational change is to occur. (For example, as the administrator in the Hemmingford case study becomes aware of a gap between the expected and actual revenues generated by each physician, he also becomes aware of the need for the organization to close this gap.)

A problem identified during the evaluation stage should be carefully analyzed to determine which factors affect the problem. For example, a health center may identify a problem with productivity, attributing it to the failure of a provider to see enough patients. However, other factors, such as fees and scheduling, also should be examined. Only after the actual cause has been determined can the appropriate response be initiated.

The evaluation stage should indicate the depth of change required to resolve the problem and whether the problem can be resolved by the current leadership. The need for a major change increases the likelihood that new leadership also is needed, since the current leadership may have strong feelings of loyalty, interests and obligations that can render them ineffective in promoting major organizational change.

Initiation

The initiation stage begins when the decision for change has been accepted by the person—typically the center administrator—who is responsible for managing the change process. In this stage, alternative strategies for problem resolution, their accompanying levels of intervention and the availability of resources must be assessed.

The depth of individuals' emotional involvement in the change process can be a central factor in choosing an appropriate level of intervention (Harrison, 1974). Strategies involving more formal and public aspects of role behavior (such as charges for patient visits) often are less costly, demand fewer skills on the part of the administrator and are more predictable in outcome than are strategies focusing on the more personal and private aspects of the individual or on interpersonal relationships (such as the amount of time spent by a physician on patient visits).

The level of intervention required by a particular strategy, the manager's ability to implement that level of intervention and the resources available often will determine the strategy selected to resolve a problem. Harrison classifies five levels of intervention: (a) attempts to alter roles; (b) attempts to alter performance; (c) attempts to alter task process; (d) attempts to alter interpersonal relationships; and (e) attempts to alter intrapersonal awareness.

Level One: Attempts to Alter Roles. This strategy involves the redistribution of tasks and resources and the relative power attached to various roles in the organization. Specifically, the tasks that need to be accomplished are determined and then distributed among various roles.

Level Two: Attempts to Alter Performance. Here, the administrator is concerned more with what an individual is able and likely to achieve professionally than with the individual's internal values. The related strategy is limited to the observable, such as setting performance goals and evaluating the individual's success or failure in attaining those goals. Direct attempts to influence performance may be made through the application of rewards and punishments.

Level Three: Attempts to Alter Task Process. This strategy focuses on how an individual organizes and conducts his or her work and how the individual's work style affects others in the organization. This includes such factors as delegating or reserving authority, communicating or withholding information and collaborating or competing with others on work-related issues. Intervention at this level attempts to change work behavior and working relationships and frequently involves bargaining or negotiating between groups and individuals.

Level Four: Attempts to Alter Interpersonal Relationships. This strategy focuses on the quality of human relationships within the organization. Direct interventions attempt to change the way individuals perceive, feel and think about one another. Examples of intervention methods include sensitivity and interpersonal growth training.

Level Five: Attempts to Alter Intrapersonal Awareness. Here the emphasis is on the individual's attitudes, values and conflicts regarding his or her own functioning and identity. Intervention efforts attempt to increase the range of experiences individuals can use to cope with problems. Individual and group therapy illustrate this approach.

The first three intervention levels are used most often by health center administrators because they tend to be less costly and more predictable in outcome. The last two levels rarely are used because the time and skill required to manage these interventions often surpass the training or experience of the administrator and because the external resources available for implementing them often are limited and costly.

The resources available to the health center are a second important factor in the selection of alternative strategies for problem resolution. The use of existing financial resources to resolve a specific problem may hamper other planned activities. Alternatively, seeking external financial resources may engender dependency on and scrutiny from the funding agency.

The time and organizational level at which a selected strategy is initially implemented have implications for the long-term effectiveness of the change. Dalton (1974) suggests that one of the most important conditions for the successful initiation of change is a sense of tension or perceived need for change among those who are targeted for change. Wieland and Ullrich (1976) contend that the effectiveness of program change may be enhanced by selecting the more powerful and cohesive units as the starting point. These units would serve as models and create pressures for other units to change, thus spreading change throughout the organization via a diffusion process.

Implementation

During the implementation stage, the impact of change on the organization becomes apparent. How individuals perceive the change and its impact on the organization depends upon the depth and extent of the intervention required to introduce and effect the change. It is during the implementation stage that conflict is most likely to surface as uncertainties about old and new procedures or personnel become obvious. The extent to which management has structured the change effort will act to either inhibit or increase conflict. Highly structured and well-planned change may provide some degree of security and reduce interpersonal conflict; it also may create an insensitivity to feedback (Wieland and Ullrich, 1976). This is not to say that conflict is inherently bad for an organization. Conflict can identify problems likely to arise in the future and may provide valuable feedback for adjusting the implementation plan to organizational realities. On the other hand, poor conflict management can lead to uncontrollable organizational responses.

Change strategies touch different aspects of the individual, groups and the organization as a whole and may produce resistance of various kinds and intensities. Change strategies require differing kinds and levels of commitment on the part of organizational members if they are to succeed, and they demand differing levels of skills and abilities on the part of the person carrying out the change.

Resistance to change is most likely to occur during the implementation stage but may develop at any point in the process of organizational change. Hage (1980) offers three explanations for resistance to change. The *vested interest* explanation holds that small power groups, especially when a substantial gap in power exists between these groups and other participants in the organization, perceive a greater threat from potential change and perceive all change as a response to a crisis situation. (The attitude of the emergency room physicians in the Montgomery County Hospital case study illustrates this type of resistance.)

The *capacity for change* explanation asserts that tolerance for change depends on prior experience with change. Individuals who have never experienced change are more resistant to current or future changes. Resistance of this type is most likely found under conditions of planned change (change without crisis). Since many health centers are relatively new organizations, there is little chance that either the board members or staff members have dealt with prior change in the organization. Therefore, when change does occur in these new organizations, the level of resistance may be high simply because those involved have not yet developed a capacity for change.

Finally, the *cost-benefit* explanation weighs the cost of change to an individual, role or program within an organization against the collective benefits to the organization resulting from that change. This resistance can occur under either crisis or planned conditions. Again, health centers in their early years are slow to develop a collective identity, and change can only be viewed from the individual's personal perspective; that is, whether the proposed change will affect the individual—rather than the organization—positively or negatively. During these early years, organizational members tend to assume that change that benefits individuals will benefit the organization as a whole. (In the Cape Meares case study, for example, the nurse/administrator is unable to see that changes are necessary for the survival of the health center. She identifies so strongly with the organization that her individual, or personal, perspective overshadows her organizational perspective.)

Routinization

The routinization stage of organizational change represents the point at which change will be rejected or accepted and, subsequently, consolidated. In this stage, roles and functions of personnel are recast and institutionalized as the demands and expectations of both the organization and its individuals converge. Management strategy must include an information feedback process that heightens acceptability. Tolerance for a moderate pace of change is more likely to be necessary in rural centers than in urban centers because resources for effecting the change may be more difficult to locate. The length of time required for an organization to arrive at the routinization stage depends upon the scope and nature of the problem that precipitated the change and the selected level of intervention.

The Life Cycle of an Organization

The process of organizational change can be viewed as a life cycle that relates to both the growth and aging of the organization as new information is obtained. Lippitt and Schmidt (1967) have developed a life-cycle concept that can be applied to health care delivery organizations. Figures 1 through 3 illustrate this adaptation in terms of three organizational life-cycle stages: (1) initial program stage; (2) middle operating stage; and (3) advanced operating stage. Each stage in turn consists of an early and a late phase.

Certain issues and needs must be addressed at each stage in the cycle if the organization is to remain viable. The extent to which these issues and needs are appropriately managed determines the extent to which the organization achieves its goals. Different management skills are required at each stage to bring the organization successfully through the cycle. Because different management skills are required at each stage, problem resolution at one stage does not automatically mean that the organization will be able to resolve problems at a later stage. The manager must either possess or develop skills appropriate to each stage, or the organization must seek a manager who does possess the necessary skills.

Management skills can be broadly classified into three categories: technical, human and conceptual. Hersey and Blanchard (1972) define these skills as follows:

☐ *Technical Skill.* Ability to use knowledge, methods, techniques and equipment necessary for the performance of specific tasks; acquired from experience, education and training.

☐ *Human Skill.* Ability and judgment in working with and through people, including an understanding of motivation and an application of effective leadership principles.

☐ *Conceptual Skill.* Ability to understand the complexities of the overall organization and where one's own operation fits into the organization. This knowledge permits one to act according to the objectives of the total organization rather than only on the basis of the goals and needs of one's own immediate group. [pp. 6-7]

The following discussion highlights the organizational concerns of each stage and those skills needed by managers to successfully pilot the organization through each stage.

The primary concerns during the initial program stage *(Figure 1)* are with organizational creation (early phase) and survival (late phase). In organizational creation, the primary emphasis is on program planning, staff selection and development and initial financing. Determination of goals and objectives, allocation of resources and implementation of services occur during this phase. The late, or survival, phase is concerned with adaptation as unfamiliar problems emerge. Events during this stage determine whether the organization will remain marginal, die or become viable.

Although all three types of management skills are needed in all of the life-cycle stages, the primary emphasis in stage 1 is the use of technical and human management skills. Managers also need some conceptual skills regarding the health care delivery system to define the direction of the organization as it moves toward the next stage. Piloting a community planning group through the planning process for a health center requires excellent technical and human skills. Technical skills are needed to create structures, procedures and policies that will provide a solid foundation for organizational growth and development. In rural areas, few resources are available for administrators lacking these skills. The Cape Meares case study illustrates a center in the first stage of development and demonstrates that learning by experience can be costly for a center.

Most rural health centers are likely to be either in this stage of development or in the process of moving into stage 2 (middle operating stage). In order to move into stage 2 successfully, many centers operated by community boards must consider recruiting new community members who can provide a fresh outlook to the organization. If new members or ideas are not introduced at this point, the center may lock itself into a recycling of old issues and ineffective solutions.

Organizational concerns in stage 2 *(see Figure 2)* focus on stability (early phase) and pride and reputation (late phase). In seeking stability, the organization begins to accommodate itself to its environment and adjust to internal operations. During this stage, differences in staff performance and expectations will become apparent and those that present problems must be resolved in order to achieve operational stability. Also, differing client expectations and needs may become apparent.

In the late phase of stage 2 (pride and reputation), the organization is concerned with establishing credibility through monitoring,

---

Figure 1 Initial Program Stage

Organizational Considerations	Early Phase	Late Phase
Critical concern	To create a new organization	To survive as a viable entity
Key issues	What to risk	What to sacrifice
Consequences if concern is not met	Frustration and inaction	Death of organization; further subsidy by "faith" capital
Result if the issue is resolved:		
Correctly	A new health care delivery system begins operating	Organization accepts realities, learns from experience, becomes viable
Incorrectly	Idea remains abstract. Service cannot develop adequately or cannot be implemented	Organization fails to adjust to realities of its environment and either dies or remains marginal
Requirements:		
Knowledge	Clearly perceived short-range objectives	The short-range objectives that need to be communicated
Skills	Ability to translate knowledge into action by self and into orders to others	Ability to communicate; ability to adjust to changing conditions
Attitudes	Belief in own ability, product and market	Faith in future
Key management decisions and problems	Services to be provided; fiscal foundation; technical procedures; political or legislative needs; organizational leadership	Focus of operation; accounting and recording procedures; recruiting and training procedures
Actions required	Define target population; determine service area; assess alternatives; make firm decisions; move with speed and flexibility; employ fluid strategy and tactics using internal and external opinions; provide for timely entrance of new services	Hire high-quality personnel; obtain financial backing at appropriate times; introduce delegation; implement basic policies with one eye on future

Figure 2 Middle Operating Stage

Organizational Considerations	Early Phase	Late Phase
Critical concern	To gain stability	To gain reputation and develop pride
Key issues	How to organize	How to review and evaluate
Consequences if concern is not met	Reactive, crisis-dominated organization; opportunistic rather than self-directing attitudes and policies	Difficulty in attracting good personnel and clients; inappropriate, overly aggressive and distorted image-building
Result if the issue is resolved:		
Correctly	Organization develops efficiency and strength but retains flexibility to change	Organization's reputation reinforces efforts to improve quality of service
Incorrectly	Organization overextends itself and returns to survival stage or establishes stabilizing patterns that block future flexibility	Organization places more effort on image-creation than on service quality or builds an image that misrepresents its true capability
Requirements:		
Knowledge	Predicting relevant factors and making long-range plans	Planning; understanding goals
Skills	Ability to translate planning knowledge into communicable objectives	Facility in allowing others a voice in decision making; involving others in decision making and obtaining commitments from them; communicating objectives to clients
Attitudes	Trust in other members of organization	Interest in clients
Key management decisions and problems	Strategic planning; appropriate responses to new competition; technological matters; internal reward system for personnel; basic public relations policies	Increasing the quality of services; escalating the flow of health education information to the service area
Actions required	Take more aggressive action in marketplace; use systematic plans and objective-setting; train personnel for future needs; promote image-building and external contacts	Meet special client needs; update policies and philosophy; concentrate on posture and image, both internal and external; assure sound financial foundation

evaluating and strategic planning. Reputation of the organization must be a major administrative concern since the "new" organization in the community is being transformed into a "regular" community entity. The organization's destiny depends more on its normal, daily performance than on opening-day activities or publicity. The Hemmingford and Tehama County Department of Health Services case studies illustrate health centers entering this middle-operating phase.

Problems encountered during stage 2 typically require human skills on the part of the administrator. Conceptual skills will become more necessary as the organization begins to move into the third stage. Although technical skills will be needed by the administrator, other staff members should be developing and using these skills in stage 2, since the administrator will be spending more time on personnel management, strategic planning and external organizational and community relations—activities that emphasize human skills. This transition from technical to human and emerging conceptual skills may be very difficult for rural health center administrators. Often, they have only recently become accustomed to and comfortable with the technical skills required in stage 1 and are reluctant to deal with issues touching upon the individuals within the organization. However, conceptual skills are needed to see beyond the individual and sometimes isolated nature of events and achieve a broader organizational view. This is difficult in any management situation and especially in a small organization in a rural area.

In stage 3, or the advanced operating stage *(Figure 3)*, organizations are concerned during the early phase with achieving uniqueness and adaptability and during the late phase with the organization's contribution to society. The early phase entails significant risk for the organization as it begins to diversify and expand. During the late phase, the organization becomes institutionalized and respected as a part of the community structure. Once a health center reaches this stage, external threats to its existence will be countered by community support.

At this point, managers must possess and use conceptual skills. Unless the manager understands how the organization fits into the larger community, the health center will remain or become an isolated entity rather than an integrated, permanent part of that community.

Certain issues and needs must be addressed at each stage in the organizational life cycle. The extent to which those issues and needs are appropriately managed determines the extent to which the organization will achieve stability and long-range viability. Managing the organization's resources toward long-range viability can be viewed conceptually as a sequence of decisions and actions that occur in

Figure 3 Advanced Operating Stage

Organizational Considerations	Early Phase	Late Phase
Critical concern	To achieve uniqueness and adaptability	To contribute to society
Key issues	Whether and how to change	Whether and how to share services
Consequences if concern is not met	Unnecessarily defensive or competitive attitudes; diffusion of energy; loss of most creative personnel	Possible lack of public respect and appreciation; loss of clientele
Result if the issue is resolved:		
Correctly	Organization changes to take better advantage of its unique capability and provides growth opportunities for its personnel	Organization gains public respect and appreciation as an institution contributing to society
Incorrectly	Organization develops too narrowly to ensure secure future, fails to discover its uniqueness and focuses efforts on inappropriate areas, or develops a paternalistic stance that inhibits growth	Organization may be accused of lack of public concern
Requirements:		
Knowledge	Understanding on part of policy team of how others should set own objectives and of how to manage sub-units of the organization	General management understanding of the larger objectives of organization and of society
Skills	Ability to teach others to plan; proficiency in integrating plans of sub-units into objectives and resources of organization	Ability to apply own organization and resources to the problems of the larger community
Attitudes	Self-confidence	Sense of responsibility to society
Key management decisions and problems	Internal audit of resources and limitations; policies to develop balance in operations	Scope of community service
Actions required	Select and promote one special service or range of services; increase delegation; provide for more effective communications, including upward flow of ideas	Broaden commitment in community (health education); concentrate on long-range direction; assess internal direction in relation to total environment

stages, have sequential relationships and demand differing information sets and skills. Mastering these stages and applying appropriate management skills represent a challenge—indeed a requirement—for managers in any setting.

Strategic Planning

Strategic planning is the iterative process of assessing the organization's current and future environments and its operating and structural characteristics; examining strengths, weaknesses, threats and opportunities in light of its environments and characteristics; and then selecting organizational strategies that match organizational goals with organizational constraints and opportunities (Hofer and Schendel, 1978).

Strategic planning is both a management tool and a process that directs an organization's attention to the future. It helps the organization adapt to change and determine the most appropriate direction for movement through the organizational life cycle. While program planning is directed at establishing the organization and guiding the initial operational period (one to three years), strategic planning is directed at adapting the existing organization to meet the challenges of the future. Unless an organization uses some form of strategic or long-range planning, organizational adaptation is likely to be haphazard and crisis-oriented, resulting in short-range solutions at the potential expense of long-range viability.

Strategic planning consists of evaluating the current state of the environment and the organization, predicting the future environment and identifying *broadly* how the organization can best "fit" into that environment. Implementation consists of identifying *specifically* what must be done to achieve an organizational/environmental fit and attempting to implement actions accordingly. The two processes overlap, since strategic planning forms the basis for developing specific plans during the implementation stage.

Some strategic planning models consider implementation to be part of the model itself (Hofer and Schendel, 1978). Others consider it a management control process separate from strategic planning (Anthony, 1965). Implementation is viewed in this chapter as a management control process in order to emphasize how strategic planning and implementation differ in focus and the importance of each in achieving long-range viability.

Strategic Planning Process

The strategic planning process presented in this chapter is a modification of Hofer and Schendel's model. The first step in the process is an internal assessment, an examination of the organization's existing goals, objectives and policies. As in many organizations, the health center's existing goals and the strategies used to achieve those goals may not be sound, fully understood or agreed upon given changes in both the environment and organizational personnel since health center start-up. The crucial initial task in a strategic planning process therefore is to identify how organizational actors view current health center directions and operations. The administrator/manager of the health center should identify key decision makers who will be involved in the planning process, explain the process to these persons and ensure that they understand both their own roles and the importance of the process to the health center.

Decision makers should formally sanction the process before it begins. For example, if the health center is governed by a community board, that board should at least be involved throughout the process. Involvement at this early point lays the groundwork for those decisions that the board eventually must make and provides the administrator with the board's view of the organization and how the board would like to see the health center develop. Regardless of the center's organizational sponsorship, providers and community members must be represented in the strategic planning process. For hospital-sponsored or provider-sponsored centers, community representation in the strategic planning process is particularly crucial in helping to determine community needs as well as alternatives that will be acceptable if chosen for implementation. Because of their importance in any rural health center, providers should be involved early in the strategic planning process. Most strategies selected for implementation will revolve around provider roles or behaviors, and early involvement will help gain their support of the strategies selected.

An effective assessment of the center's structure and internal operations requires that all key personnel are willing to identify and constructively examine the weaknesses as well as the strengths of the center. For this reason, the internal assessment component of the strategic planning process is often the most difficult to manage. A well-designed evaluation plan from the program planning process should help by providing data on patient care programs and services, support services, organizational structure (including personnel) and finances.

The second step in the strategic planning process—an external assessment—enables a center to evaluate the logic, relevance and appropriateness of its current goals, objectives, strategies and policies in the context of the center's present and future environment. By combining the findings of the internal and external assessments, the health center can begin to understand which internal and external forces will affect it in the future.

While the external environmental assessment encompasses all factors examined during program planning, the analytic perspective differs in strategic planning. In program planning, the factors are analyzed to predict their potential effect on utilization. Strategic planning considers their actual effect on utilization and predicts their continuing and future effect. If, for example, the center's service area contains a large number of individuals aged 65 and over, program planning might address Medicare/Medicaid certification requirements and scope of coverage. In strategic planning, however, the issues to be addressed might include: which center services are not covered by Medicare/Medicaid; the extent to which Medicare/Medicaid is covering health center costs; how the center would be affected if Medicare/Medicaid reimbursement were reduced; and how continuation of the aging trend of the population will affect the health center. The real challenge in small organizations is identifying a mechanism (literature searches, interagency contacts, provider contacts, professional meetings) for obtaining data that highlights external issues and trends. External assessments often are more difficult in a small, rural organization because these organizations have a propensity for focusing on internal and/or local issues.

The third step in the strategic planning process involves comparing current health center performance, objectives and position in the environment (as identified during the internal and external assessments) with both the projected and the desired future status of the health center. The purpose of this step is to identify gaps between the current and the desired future position of the organization and then to identify action alternatives for closing those gaps.

The final step in the strategic planning process is decision making. Here, action alternatives derived from step 3 are evaluated by applying various criteria such as cost, benefits and risks to each one; the alternatives then are ranked based on the cost/benefit/risk analysis. Key decision makers must agree on the options selected for implementation, since agreement will heighten organizational commitment to the selected options. As in program planning, however, agreement may be difficult to achieve, particularly in sensitive areas. Unless managers are sensitive to the problems associated with issue resolution, the strategic planning process can collapse at this point with potentially destructive effects on the health center as an organization.

The strategic planning process may produce a redefined goal statement for the health center as a provider of services to the community. If the strategic planning process has been successful, it will identify the optimal fit between community needs and organizational constraints, capabilities and opportunities. Identification of this optimal fit is the necessary foundation for ensuring the long-range viability of the organization. The written strategic plan can be viewed as a communication tool that provides a clear statement of organizational direction and a summary of those strategies selected by the organization to help it move in that direction.

Implementation of Strategic Plans

Once appropriate organizational strategies are formulated and priorities are assigned to these strategies, specific implementation plans must be formulated and carried out. Implementation encompasses three components: action planning, actual program implementation and program control and evaluation.

Action planning entails developing a specific plan for implementing the priorities selected by decision makers in the strategic planning process. This includes identifying tasks, responsibilities and a time table for implementation, identifying a marketing strategy and establishing a budget. Although action planning is typically an administrative responsibility, rural health centers, because of their small size, could effectively use a team approach to action planning. The team should consist of those in the organization who will be performing new roles or otherwise be affected by the actions being implemented. For example, if a change from a manual to a computerized billing system is planned, the team might consist of the bookkeeper, administrator, medical director, a board member and an external computer consultant. Attracting a new service area population group might call for a team consisting of a nurse, the medical director, the administrator, a board member and an outreach or social worker. While the team approach helps reduce resistance and gain individual commitment to change, the administrator must assume responsibility for coordinating the team efforts.

Once action plans have been formulated, the programs are implemented by appropriate personnel within the organization according to the plan. During this phase, management must continue to be sensitive to resistance to change.

The final implementation step is program control and evaluation. The control and evaluation activity ensures management that program implementation is consistent with the action plan and provides the opportunity for alterations in implementation strategy before problems arise. Management also should use this opportunity to obtain and provide feedback in the organization as it continues to adapt to changing internal and external conditions.

Financial Viability

Financial viability is a key issue as a rural health center undertakes strategic planning. The long-range viability of rural primary care centers is related to and dependent on solving the long-standing problem of insufficient financing for rural health care. Financial stability is a necessary goal for centers in achieving long-range viability; for some, financial self-sufficiency is the necessary goal. Reaching financial stability and self-sufficiency may be more difficult in the future than it has been in the last decade because of decreasing federal funding support and reimbursement program limitations and reductions.

If a health center cannot achieve financial self-sufficiency under its existing structure and operation, the sponsor and/or community board will have to make a crucial decision about whether the center can afford to stay in business. Decisions to close a health center, sell it or merge with another operation are never easy to make. The leadership needs to be open to seeing the health center as a different kind of organization than the one that exists. Options such as selling the practice to an institution or providers, working with a private practice in another town or merging with a broader regional network of health centers may need to be considered. It is particularly difficult for community-owned health centers to consider options that change ownership, since board and community members often have invested a great deal of time and energy to open and maintain the health center and sometimes see a change of ownership as reducing or eliminating their participation. This need not be the case, however, if the community is clear about and can negotiate a continued role under a new structure.

Several generic environmental factors present obstacles to a health center's ability to achieve financial stability (Lichty and Zuvekas, 1980). They are:

☐ Employed residents of rural areas tend to work in low-benefit industries that provide inadequate or no health insurance for their workers. This means that workers themselves often must pay for services. Given the general low income levels in rural areas and the shortage of third-party coverage, the purchasing power of rural residents for medical care tends to be severely limited.

☐ Medicare and Medicaid policies often discriminate against rural areas and rural health centers in the following ways:

— lower reimbursement levels are provided than for the same services provided in urban areas,

— rural residents have more difficulty qualifying for Medicaid since they are more likely to live in intact families, and

— Medicaid programs are generally more restrictive in rural states.

☐ Significant services provided by the centers, including health education and screening programs and others that respond to unmet medical needs, have not been reimbursed by any paying agency.

While the terms financial self-sufficiency and financial viability are both related to long-range viability, they indicate different financing directions for health centers and different implications for long-range viability. A financially viable center is one that has obtained sufficient financial support to cover the cost of services provided. These revenues probably include subsidies from one or more external sources, including federal funding programs. A financially viable center has resources to remain in business but may not be self-sufficient. In contrast, the entire expense budget of a financially self-sufficient center is covered by revenues from direct patient or third-party payments, including Medicare and Medicaid (Feldman and others, 1978).

Many centers have achieved short-term (one to three years) financial viability during start-up by participating in demonstration grant programs. Their ability to maintain existing levels of service typically depends on the continuing availability of federal and other grant resources. When these resources are reduced, as they are expected to be during the 1980s, the centers must reduce their services, obtain or increase other sources of revenue or terminate services altogether. At the state level, financial viability is affected by Medicaid eligibility, benefit exclusion and reimbursement policies. If the political and economic climate of the early 1980s persists, the financial viability of health centers will increasingly be tied to their ability to achieve self-sufficiency through direct patient and third-party revenues.

Of the many strategic issues identified by the planning process, nearly all relate to the need for increasing center self-sufficiency. Among the key internal (operational/management) issues that relate directly to financial viability and should be considered carefully in strategic planning are: patient volume potential, market penetration, scope of services, fee setting, and billing and collection policies.

Patient Volume Potential

Each center must identify the population groups and service area that it expects or wants to serve, taking into account such factors as mobility of the population, customary practice patterns for external referrals and established utilization patterns. The volume potential includes not only those currently served, but also a larger population group that could be served if operational policies such as hours of operation, services offered and access to providers were changed. For example, several studies concluded that financial self-sufficiency is more likely to be achieved if laboratory tests are performed onsite and if center providers are able to hospitalize patients.

Market Penetration

The center must influence utilization behavior so that the needs of the service area population are translated into demands for center services. Market penetration is the process of making services and programs known to the service area population, influencing the population to use these services and programs and then retaining its loyalty. Studies demonstrate that loyalty and long-term utilization (that is, market penetration) appear to occur when a wide range of medical procedures is available and when ambulatory services are provided onsite. Continuity of service provision and of service providers also affects market penetration.

Scope of Services

The center must be able to provide a comprehensive range of services, including preventive, early diagnostic and continuing (follow-up) care. The scope of services a center can or should provide is related not only to service area factors but also to revenue potential. Health center administrators or sponsors often are faced with the conflict of providing services that will accelerate market penetration but have little reimbursement or revenue potential. In striving for long-range viability, a center must always consider the addition of revenue-producing services and maximizing options for reimbursement. In the early stages of development, it may be appropriate to offer nonreimbursable services through subsidies to accelerate market penetration and demonstrate efficacy. However, careful financial planning to cover the cost of services is necessary to avoid long-term deficit spending or the discontinuation of services.

Setting Fees

Setting fees for services is a critical policy decision for managers. If fees are set below costs, self-sufficiency may never be reached. If fees are too high, clients may go elsewhere. Many rural centers receiving federal funds have used a sliding fee scale, a viable option when subsidies are available. The gradual reduction and elimination of these subsidies, however, makes the sliding fee scale a liability for self-sufficiency if a large number of center clients are charged less than the cost of the services. Center self-sufficiency is best achieved when fees are set at cost levels.

Billing and Collection Policies

Centers must develop an effective and efficient procedure for billing and collection. A center's collection effort may well determine the success or failure of its efforts to become financially self-sufficient. Third-party payer billings, including Medicare and Medicaid, must be pursued aggressively to maintain a sufficient cash flow.

The organizational policies discussed above constitute one of many factors that influence a center's ability to achieve financial viability and self-sufficiency. Other factors include affiliations with HMOs and shared service arrangements, community circumstances, practitioner practice patterns, consumer preferences and organizational performance. Finally, staff motivation is also an important factor. Staff members must be committed and able to contribute to the center's problem solution effort. Unless the staff is committed to making the center work, there is little chance that even the best strategies will succeed (Wade and Brooks, 1979).

Summary

The external environment cannot be overlooked as a significant factor in the achievement of long-range viability for rural primary care centers. While centers should be concerned about and encourage policy makers to address external issues, centers also must accept the reality of the environment and adapt the organization's internal environment to it. The internal environment of the health center is the environment over which the health center can achieve greater control.

This chapter presented three major factors that are crucial in a center's ability to adapt to environmental conditions, both internal and external, and achieve long-range viability: program planning, organizational growth and development and strategic planning. Through careful program planning, a health center manager or sponsor can avoid wasting resources in crisis intervention and in solving problems that need not have occurred. Program planning entails assessing the environment, planning the facility, developing clear goals and objectives and continually evaluating operations.

Health center managers also must recognize organizational change and growth and be prepared to adapt. For health centers, the process of organizational change can be viewed as having four stages: evaluation, initiation, implementation and routinization. Organizational change occurs in a life cycle consisting of three stages, each with an early and a late phase: initial program stage, middle operating stage and advanced operating stage. At each stage, certain issues and needs must be addressed if the organization is to remain viable. Each stage also requires certain management skills to bring the organization successfully through the cycle.

Strategic planning is both a management tool and a process that directs an organization's attention to the future; in other words, it helps the organization determine the most appropriate direction for movement through the organizational life cycle. The model presented in this chapter consists of a three-step strategic planning process followed by a three-step implementation process.

Financial viability cannot be separated from long-range viability; if a rural health center cannot reach financial stability and/or financial self-sufficiency, it likely will not achieve long-range viability. Therefore, financial planning must be an integral part of the organization's strategic planning process. Financial viability (and self-sufficiency) is affected by both the external and internal environments. The key internal issues that should be considered in strategic planning because of their potential effect on finances are: patient volume potential, market penetration, scope of services, fee setting, and billing and collection policies.

There are no concrete formulas for success in achieving and maintaining long-range viability because organizations, including rural health centers, vary by type and size, geographic location, work force characteristics and external influences. This chapter has merely presented a framework within which center managers can identify strengths, weaknesses and opportunities for the health center. Such a framework, when combined with leadership that is analytical, flexible when identifying alternatives for program development and problem resolution and sensitive to organizational and community needs and individuals, will enable a health center to stay in business over the long-run.

References

Aiken, M., and Hage, J. The organic organization and innovation. *Sociology,* 5(1971):63.

Anthony, R.N. *Planning and Control Systems: A Framework for Analysis.* Boston: Harvard University, 1965.

Dalton, G. Influence and organizational change. In D.A. Kolb and others (eds.), *Organizational Psychology: A Book of Readings,* 2nd ed. Englewood Cliffs, NJ: Prentice-Hall, 1974.

Deniston, O.L., and Rosenstock, I.M. Evaluating health programs. *Public Health Rep.,* 85(1978):9.

Feldman, R., and others. The financial viability of rural primary health care centers. *Am. J. Public Health,* 68(1978):981.

Gurwitz, K., and Dennis, R. Lake country, Michigan: A profile of rural poverty, public health, and a plan that failed. *Public Health Rep.,* 90(1975):357.

Hage, J. *Theories of Organizations: Form, Process, and Transformation.* New York: John Wiley & Sons, 1980.

Harrison, R. Some criteria for choosing the depth of organizational intervention strategy. In D.A. Kolb and others (eds.), *Organizational Psychology: A Book of Readings,* 2nd ed. Englewood Cliffs, NJ: Prentice-Hall, 1974.

Hersey, P., and Blanchard, K.H. *Management of Organizational Behavior,* 2nd ed. Englewood Cliffs, NJ: Prentice-Hall, 1972.

Hofer, C.W., and Schendel, D. *Strategy Formulation: Analytical Concepts.* St. Paul, MN: West Publishing Co., 1978.

Hyman, H.H. *Health Planning: A Systematic Approach.* Germantown, MD: Aspen Systems Corporation, 1976.

Lichty, S.S., and Zuvekas, A. Rural health: Policies, progress, and challenge. *Urban Health,* 9(1980):26.

Lippitt, G.L., and Schmidt, W.H. Crises in a developing organization. *Harv. Bus. Rev.,* 45(1967):102.

Wade, T.L., and Brooks, E.F. *Planning and Managing Rural Health Centers.* Cambridge, MA: Ballinger Publishing Co., 1979.

Wieland, G.F., and Ullrich, R.A. *Organizations: Behavior, Design and Change.* Chicago: Richard D. Irwin, Inc., 1976.

Cases

Christine P. Howell
Rosemary L. Summers

Ms. Howell, principal author of the case studies, is communications manager, the Hospital Research and Educational Trust, Chicago.

Ms. Summers, contributing author of the case studies, was casebook coordinator for the Innovations in Ambulatory Primary Care project.

[While the case studies are based on actual experience of the IAPC sites, the site names, locations, names of individuals and other factors have been fictionalized and should not be attributed to any particular site. Any similarities to other organizations, locales or individuals are purely coincidental.]

6
C. T. Meyer Hospital

C. T. Meyer Hospital

In July 1977, Nick Ryerson was employed by the administrator of C.T. Meyer Hospital of Morgan Hill, Maine. His assignment was to develop two nearby rural ambulatory primary care health centers that had been struggling for years to become viable community health care resources. Mr. Ryerson was a recent graduate of George Washington University, Washington, D.C., where he was awarded a master's degree in health administration. He was familiar with health care delivery in small communities because he had worked at two rural hospitals and for a public health department in a small New England town. Mr. Ryerson also was familiar with the Morgan Hill region, having spent many summers there at his family's vacation home.

Mr. Ryerson had conducted a feasibility study of primary care in the Morgan Hill area as one project for his master's degree. It was while conducting this study that Mr. Ryerson first met Dr. Timothy White, a practicing physician in the area for 30 years. The professional and personal relationship that developed between the two men was the key to Mr. Ryerson's 1977 appointment at C.T. Meyer Hospital.

Mr. Ryerson was hired by the 40-bed nonprofit hospital to administer a $148,000, two-year grant* that had been awarded to the hospital to stimulate and redevelop ambulatory primary care resources in the rural environs around Morgan Hill, beginning with a rejuvenation of two community health centers—one in the village of Jackson and the other in the village of Charlotte *(Figure 1)*.

Upon assuming his post, Mr. Ryerson encountered a confusing and apparently conflicting situation. Mr. Ryerson said, "When I came, what I basically had was a bank book with the grant money deposited and the grant application. I tried to figure out from the grant application what the objectives of the hospital were and how they related to the goals of the sponsoring community groups but got pretty confused. In the meantime, the two health centers were in operation, had been in some fashion for a number of years and had no idea what an administrator was for."

Mr. Ryerson's initial confusion stemmed from several factors. The

---

*The grant was awarded by the Hospital Research and Educational Trust through funding from the W. K. Kellogg Foundation.

160

Figure 1 Green County, Maine

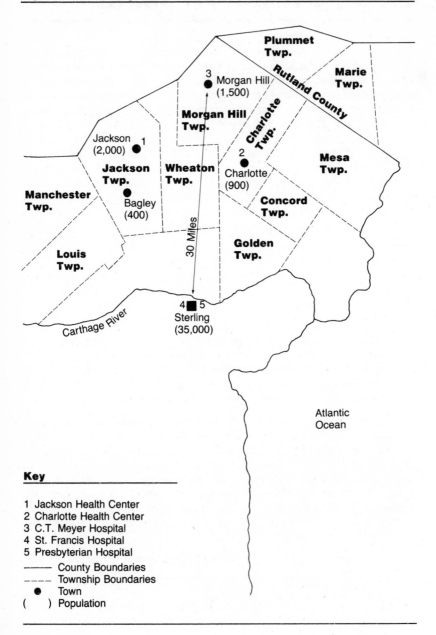

Key

1 Jackson Health Center
2 Charlotte Health Center
3 C.T. Meyer Hospital
4 St. Francis Hospital
5 Presbyterian Hospital

——— County Boundaries
- - - - Township Boundaries
● Town
(   ) Population

hospital's grant application, written almost entirely by Dr. White, contained only vague generalities about the hospital's plans and objectives in using the grant funds (see *Exhibit)*. The two sponsoring community groups referred to in the grant application were in fact three groups, two of which were at odds with each other. The communities were uninformed and skeptical about the hospital's plans for the health centers. The two health centers were in a state of financial and administrative disarray. And the C.T. Meyer Hospital had been beset with low occupancy rates and financial problems for the past five years *(Figure 2)*.

Dr. White

Through his association with Dr. White, Nick Ryerson realized that the major problems with the grant application stemmed from Dr. White and his style. Dr. White was a poetic visionary with a zest for life, strong interpersonal skills and an ability to transform his visions into reality. In Dr. White's own words, he had made some progress "with the aid of some wonderful people, but the effort was characterized by unorganized travail and held together with baling wire and friction tape. I had a good policy manual (The Golden Rule), but it lacked structural detail. I needed someone to fill in that detail." While Mr. Ryerson could use Dr. White as a sounding board and a source of encouragement—which he did often in his early months—he could not rely on Dr. White for answers to organizational questions.

Mr. Ryerson was also aware that Dr. White was a highly respected and dynamic force in community health care. During the 1940s, Dr. White had encouraged wealthy shipper C.T. Meyer to build C. T. Meyer Hospital as part of a four-facility system after a state survey had identified a serious shortage of hospital facilities in the smaller towns along the Maine coastline. Dr. White served as chief of the medical staff at C.T. Meyer Hospital for many years, and in the early 1960s, he had joined with the other three Morgan Hill physicians to form the Morgan Hill Medical Group (MHMG). This corporation became the primary provider of medical care in the region and comprised the medical staff of the C.T. Meyer Hospital.

The health centers in the villages of Jackson and Charlotte existed primarily because of Dr. White's efforts. Although each center had originated years earlier as a local community effort to attract private physicians, the health centers that existed at the time Mr. Ryerson was hired were the result of Dr. White joining forces with the community groups and arranging for the MHMG physicians to practice at them. The hospital's act of seeking a grant for the health centers—a grant for which the community boards operating the health centers were

Figure 2 Financial and Utilization Data, 1972–1977–C.T. Meyer Hospital of Morgan Hill

Financial Data:	10/1/72–9/30/73	10/1/73–9/30/74	10/1/74–9/30/75	10/1/75–12/31/76	1/1/77–12/31/77
Operating revenues:					
Patient service revenues	$ 800,921	$1,034,762	$1,352,926	$2,139,264	$1,727,011
*Contractual allowances and uncollectible accounts	(715)	35,264	(102,901)	(441,693)	360,555
Other operating revenue	14,722	19,956	19,173	36,730	26,156
Total operating revenue	814,928	1,089,982	1,269,198	1,734,301	1,392,612
Operating expenses:					
Nursing	345,189	403,221	418,645	556,111	439,293
Other professional services	217,790	298,716	392,654	602,862	440,659
General services	173,674	204,415	268,340	325,865	274,479
Administrative services	162,775	225,448	266,977	391,842	332,190
Provision for depreciation & amortization	74,460	78,709	79,730	99,852	83,345
Total operating expenses	973,888	1,210,509	1,426,346	1,976,532	1,569,966
Loss from operations	(158,960)	(120,527)	(157,148)	(242,231)	(177,354)
Nonoperating revenue:					
Unrestricted gifts & bequests	14,427	53,645	27,123	121,159	38,934
Investment income	2,197	3,652	4,895	7,910	7,215
Gain on sale of securities	-0-	-0-	-0-	-0-	-0-
Adjustment of prior year pension costs	-0-	-0-	-0-	-0-	37,832
Grant income	-0-	-0-	-0-	-0-	-0-
Total nonoperating revenue	16,624	57,297	32,018	129,069	83,981
Excess of revenues (expense)	(142,336)	(63,230)	(125,130)	(113,162)	(93,373)
Fund balance at beginning of period	1,414,544	1,340,076	1,276,846	1,159,671	1,046,509
Equity in assets of extension clinics	-0-	-0-	-0-	-0-	-0-
Fund balance at end of year	$1,340,076	$1,276,846	$1,159,671	$1,046,509	$953,136
* (Provision for uncollectible accounts	10,500	33,500	35,000	97,800	75,293)
Utilization Data:					
Admissions	1,178	1,113	1,260	1,351	1,482
Census (ave. daily)	23	30	28	35	36
Occupancy rate	65.7%	75.0%	62.2%	70.0%	72.0%

ineligible because they were not incorporated—was due in large measure to Dr. White's past involvement with the communities combined with his influence at the hospital.

As he became more familiar with Dr. White and with the C.T. Meyer Hospital, Mr. Ryerson gathered that Dr. White's prominent role in the health care community had evolved, at least in part, from his diplomacy in dealing with Roger Hawley, C.T. Meyer's administrator for the past 30 years. Dr. White once intimated that Mr. Hawley's time commitment to the hospital in recent years was inadequate. It seemed to Mr. Ryerson that Dr. White typically managed to circumvent Mr. Hawley or bring him around to supporting his own views.

From everything he knew about Dr. White, Mr. Ryerson felt that, while he would be of little assistance in practical matters, he could be a valuable ally in dealing with the two communities, the hospital and the medical group. However, since Dr. White planned to retire before the end of the year, Mr. Ryerson wondered if it would be wise to rely on him.

The Plans for the Health Center

When Dr. White wrote the grant application with assistance from Mr. Hawley, he believed that the grant funds could be used to solve several problems. Revitalizing the two floundering health centers would provide residents of the traditionally medically underserved communities with a reliable and stable source of local primary medical care. Success of the centers also would resolve another of Dr. White's concerns—the impact of his retirement on the community. His retirement would mean the loss of a general practitioner to the patients he had served for 30 years; his absence from the ranks of the MHMG (the area's major and almost sole provider of primary and speciality care for nearly 20 years), for which he had served as organizer, recruiter and provider; and the loss of a physician preceptor to the health centers.

Dr. White realized that, in order for the hospital to consent to seeking the grant for the health centers, the hospital would need to benefit as well. Dr. White pointed out to administrator Hawley that using the grant money to bolster the health centers would provide a distinct benefit to the hospital by helping to resolve its financial difficulties. The grant money was the means to start a regional primary care network in the area through which the C.T. Meyer Hospital could expand its referral base and attract new physicians, thereby improving its occupancy rates and financial position.

The regionalization concept described in the hospital's grant application was based on the premise that the existing community groups in Jackson and Charlotte would form a regional corporation whose board would oversee the two primary care centers. Once the regional group was incorporated for tax and funding purposes, the hospital intended to cease its involvement in health center operations.

Mr. Ryerson first heard about these plans during his initial job interviews and supported the regionalization idea for several reasons. First, a regional board would permit efficiencies of scale not otherwise possible—in cost, service provision and administration. Second, the existence of a viable primary care network corresponded to the hospital's need for higher utilization and would help in recruiting new medical personnel to the area. Third, Mr. Ryerson viewed a regional primary care network as the first step toward creating a broader network that would extend beyond the 11-township service area. Fourth, he knew that a regional network would help prepare the hospital, as well as the entire region, for a growing federal trend in health resources: areawide planning.

While Mr. Ryerson supported the idea of a regional network, he questioned the hospital's intention to disassociate itself from the health centers once the regional corporation was formed. Mr. Ryerson believed that this decision was premature and that alternative arrangements might prove more advantageous.

Ryerson's Initial Steps

Mr. Ryerson's first step in his new position was to thoroughly analyze the situation to determine what problems the health centers had encountered in the past; how knowledgeable and committed the community groups were; and how the hospital's financial situation might affect his ability to complete the task before him.

The C.T. Meyer Hospital

C.T. Meyer Hospital of Morgan Hill was one of two remaining hospitals and a long-term care facility owned and operated by Coastal Hospitals, Inc., a multi-institutional system founded in 1947 by Charles Tracy Meyer. The system was administered by Roger Hawley, who also served as chief executive officer of each of the three facilities. Mr. Hawley was located at Coastal Hospitals' Rutland, Maine, facility. Like the other facilities, C. T. Meyer Hospital had its own governing board and an onsite nurse/superintendent responsible for day-to-day operations. Rachel Blum had held that post for 20 years.

Mr. Ryerson learned that, since 1972, C.T. Meyer Hospital had been able to stay afloat through endowment funds donated to the Coastal Hospitals facilities by the C.T. Meyer Foundation. The foundation contributed $750,000 to the C.T. Meyer Hospital of Morgan Hill from 1972 to 1977. In 1977 alone, the hospital sustained an operating loss of $177,354.

Data that Mr. Ryerson collected from hospital discharge records for the previous year showed a low utilization of the hospital by residents of the ambulatory care service area *(Figure 3)*. The hospital's low penetration in the service area was an indication to Mr. Ryerson of underlying problems between the hospital and the surrounding community that could hamper the success of the health centers and the plan for a regional network.

Mr. Ryerson attributed some of the hospital's problems to its management organization and style. Mr. Hawley administered the hospital from a distance, was at the hospital only about once a month and acted more as a figurehead than an involved chief executive. Growing regulatory activity in the state during recent years was usurping Mr. Hawley's time and attention, leaving less time for administering the Coastal facilities. C.T. Meyer Hospital of Morgan Hill operated without well-defined goals and objectives and had taken no visible steps to reverse its deteriorating financial situation.

Through contacts with leaders in the community, Mr. Ryerson

Figure 3 Degree of Penetration of C.T. Meyer Hospital of Morgan Hill by Ambulatory Care Service Area Township*

Township	Population	Discharge from CTMH-MH Per 1,000 Population	Degree of Penetration
Morgan Hill	3,515	119.77	99.31%
Mesa	1,794	11.14	9.23%
Jackson	4,021	50.98	42.27%
Plummet	1,016	98.42	81.61%
Manchester	1,749	6.86	5.68%
Golden	3,972	3.27	2.71%
Wheaton	1,926	52.41	43.45%
Marie	643	15.55	12.89%
Charlotte	1,754	75.83	62.87%
Louis	1,548	12.90	10.69%
Concord	1,355	16.23	13.45%

*Prepared August 1977 based on data for period 7/76-7/77.

substantiated his theory that there were underlying problems between the hospital and service area residents. Numerous individuals voiced dissatisfaction with the quality and cost of hospital services. The mayor of Jackson expressed this dissatisfaction by stating: "I didn't have much faith in their laboratory and x-ray facilities, especially considering their cost to users. We were better off going to Sterling."

The Morgan Hill Medical Group (MHMG) was another source of negative feelings about the C.T. Meyer Hospital. Residents of both Jackson and Charlotte had been dissatisfied with the arrangements for physician resources at the health centers that were worked out between Dr. White, the other four MHMG physicians and the respective community advisory boards. Under the arrangements, which already had been abandoned at Charlotte, the MHMG physicians had agreed to staff the two centers on a part-time, rotating basis. Community complaints that had surfaced as a result of these arrangements were: lack of physician continuity; the limitations of part-time services; difficulties in relating to the MHMG providers, several of whom were foreign medical graduates; and a perceived lack of commitment on the part of the MHMG providers other than Dr. White.

The physician assistant at the Jackson center under Dr. White's preceptorship related the following impressions to Mr. Ryerson about the MHMG's reception in Jackson: "The physicians were not much help. I think it was primarily a language problem. They were both foreign and were competent physicians, but they had a language problem. Also, they were too 'big city' medicine; for example, if someone suffered from hypertension, they would do a complete workup, IVP, chest x-ray, renal studies—you name it. That was OK until the farmer got the first bill and it equaled his entire month's milk check; he would never come back." Because the MHMG also comprised the medical staff for the C.T. Meyer Hospital and was located there, community reaction to the MHMG as physician providers for the health centers extended to the hospital, exacerbating the hospital's already negative image in the community.

All of these factors—negative feelings about the hospital, the history of physician shortages in the rural areas and the inability to establish the health centers as a viable resource—had combined to produce a reliance on medical services in Sterling, a town 30 miles from Morgan Hill. The C.T. Meyer Hospital and the two health centers had been unable to reverse that pattern.

Mr. Ryerson concluded that what he discovered about the hospital and its position in the community posed several significant implications to the task facing him. He would need to rely on the resources and reputation of the C.T. Meyer Hospital to attract physician and other resources to the rural health centers. Yet the hospital had a poor reputation, its solvency was questionable and both the hospital and the community health centers had struggled unsuccessfully for years to attract a stable medical personnel supply. Given the shortage of physician resources, Mr. Ryerson knew he would have to at least consider using the MHMG to staff one or both health centers, yet community receptivity to the MHMG had already proven to be a problem. Mr. Ryerson also would have to overcome the population's orientation to Sterling services, yet some of the causes seemed beyond his control. At the same time, Mr. Ryerson's concept of regionalization implied that he would need to find some way to utilize the higher level of services (secondary and tertiary) available in Sterling and not at the C.T. Meyer Hospital, which was a primary care inpatient facility.

Before Mr. Ryerson could address these dilemmas, a series of events took place that altered his role at the hospital. It began when Mr. Hawley visited Mr. Ryerson in his office at the hospital to ask him to conduct a study of how Maine regulations were affecting the hospital's costs. Mr. Ryerson agreed to take on the task "because the project sounded interesting and might give me better insight into the problems at the hospital that I knew were going to impact on my job of administering the health centers and forming the building blocks of a regional network."

In the process of conducting the study, Mr. Ryerson experienced his first involvement with the hospital's department managers:

> I soon found myself getting more and more involved in hospital matters beyond the ambulatory care project. Once I got to know them, department heads began seeking me out for advice and intervention in hospital matters unrelated to my assigned job. It seems that they were dissatisified with decision making under Rachel Blum, the nurse/superintendent. They viewed me as someone who had access to both White and Hawley and an 'outsider' who could serve as a mediator between them [the managers] and Rachel Blum. They were approaching me to help them out with problems that ranged from staffing conflicts to servicing and replacing equipment. In one month, I spent half my time on hospital activities that bore no direct relationship to the health centers.

The Communities

The health centers in Jackson and Charlotte had been formed through the combined initiative of the respective communities and Dr. White. When the communities were unsuccessful in attracting or retaining private-practice physicians, Dr. White had proposed setting up community advisory organizations capable of raising money to back the effort and using the MHMG to provide medical care. In both instances, Dr. White and the supervisors of the four or five surrounding townships had formed organizations to raise start-up money and oversee the centers: the Palowee River Regional Health Services (PRRHS) in Charlotte and the Jackson Area Health Services (JAHS) in Jackson. From then until Mr. Ryerson's appointment, the health centers had managed to survive by means of revenue (taxes and CETA funds) allocated to them by the township supervisors and the efforts of Dr. White and the other organizers to provide whatever assistance they could to the health centers' operation.

Mr. Ryerson's talks with community leaders suggested that the tradition of community initiative and involvement in the health centers had engendered a strong sense of self-interest and community ownership that might run counter to the hospital's plans for the centers. Mr. Ryerson's theory was borne out by the recent formation of a splinter group in Jackson to circumvent the hospital's plans for the Jackson township's health center.

Under the leadership of the mayor of Jackson (a long-time political rival of Guy Jordan, the Jackson township supervisor who had organized the Jackson Area Health Services with Dr. White), a group of concerned citizens organized the Jackson Improvement Association (JIA). Those joining the mayor in forming the JIA were already disgruntled with the Jackson health center, the MHMG and the C.T. Meyer Hospital and wanted no part of a health center that had even closer ties to the hospital. To the JIA, the most objectionable element of the hospital's plan under the grant was the relocation of the Jackson health center to Bagley, 10 miles from Jackson but in the same township. The health center would continue to serve Jackson, but the rationale behind moving it was that there were no adequate existing facilities in Jackson, and Bagley was in the middle of the health center's service area. In formulating that element of the plan, Dr. White had obtained the consent of Guy Jordan and the other Jackson township supervisors. The board of supervisors had passed a resolution to make a vacant school in Bagley available for relocating the health center and to commit tax money to renovate it.

Jackson's mayor and six other residents organized the JIA as a totally separate initiative to attract private physicians to Jackson by constructing a modern, well-equipped facility. Within six months, the group had incorporated, obtained a preliminary land commitment for the facility across from a new senior citizen's housing project in Jackson, developed plans for a new building that they planned to sell or lease to a physician or physician group who agreed to settle there, interviewed several physician candidates and raised $60,000 from 1,000 Jackson residents who supported their effort.

Mr. Ryerson admired the determination of the JIA and was impressed with the success it had achieved in only six months. His concern about the JIA was the threat it posed to the immediate goal of establishing a successful Jackson/Bagley health center and to the ultimate goal of regionalization. If the JIA's efforts succeeded, the physician practice would compete with the health center as well as conflict with Mr. Ryerson's efforts to establish a regional framework.

Despite the problems the JIA presented, Mr. Ryerson realized the organization had certain strengths that could prove useful and perhaps necessary to his own efforts—if those strengths could be redirected. Among them were the JIA's strong organizational ability, its access to resources and its influence in the Jackson community. In addition, the JIA had already begun forging a link with St. Francis Hospital in Sterling, which had tentatively agreed to provide educational programming for the JIA's physician facility. Mr. Ryerson saw this initial link with St. Francis as a potentially useful tool in forging an areawide regional network beyond the scope of the C.T. Meyer Hospital. He also was aware that the other major hospital in Sterling controlled all the ambulatory care sites in and around Sterling. Therefore, if St. Francis intended to expand into ambulatory care, it would have to do so in the rural areas of the county.

The Health Centers

Mr. Ryerson's examination of records and his contacts with center staff to learn about the health centers identified a series of problems—financial, utilization, manpower, facility and administrative. He felt that most of the problems could not be dealt with in isolation because they were closely related to community attitudes that had evolved over time. Mr. Ryerson reported:

> When I examined the health centers, I found that each had its own way—and not a very sophisticated way—of doing just about everything. Basically, they were managing to get by because of the involvement of Dr. White and the Morgan Hill Medical Group, combined with some community people who were lending helping hands. The Charlotte center's

accounting system was a good illustration of the make-shift methods they employed. Township supervisor Rod Gardner's secretary performed the bookkeeping: she had the checkbook in her kitchen, she would write the checks and I would go over and sign them. She did a good job of keeping the books, but you certainly couldn't use them for reporting to third parties.

Each center was failing to collect between $1,500 and $2,000 a month in patient charges. Mr. Ryerson attributed the overall financial picture to the health centers' lack of incorporation, which severely limited their access to funding, and to the low utilization patterns caused by years of unreliable service and the image of the health centers in the community. As of mid-1977, the average combined utilization of the two centers was 420 patients per month—195 at Charlotte and 225 at Jackson. This represented less than two percent of the total service area population.

Although Mr. Ryerson knew that utilization would have to begin showing increases immediately, he had little hope the centers would reach the service projections described in the grant application. Like the remainder of the application, Mr. Ryerson thought Dr. White's projections of patient utilization for the health centers were somewhat ambiguous and overstated. The grant application had projected that the health centers would be serving a total of 8,800 patients out of the combined service area population of 25,400 after the first year under the grant and 11,160 patients after the second year. The projections apparently had failed to consider some of the factors that Mr. Ryerson believed would limit the health centers' ability to attract patients: the geographic dispersion of the population, the lack of transportation systems, severe winter road conditions, the population's apparent lack of confidence in the health centers and, most importantly, the population's orientation toward seeking primary care in Sterling. Mr. Ryerson felt that if he was held accountable—by the hospital, the grantor or the communities—for achieving the degree of penetration described in the grant, his position soon would be in jeopardy.

Inseparable from the problem of attracting patients to the centers was the problem of attracting physicians to the area—physicians who would both engender confidence among the patient population and who would stay in the area. For several years now, the MHMG had been able to attract only foreign medical specialists who remained in the Morgan Hill area for two years at most. Mr. Ryerson's ability to increase utilization of the health centers would depend in large part on the quality and quantity of physician resources he could muster.

At the time Mr. Ryerson was hired, only the Jackson health center was utilizing the part-time services of the MHMG. Jackson had a full-time physician assistant, recruited by Dr. White and working under his preceptorship. With Dr. White's retirement, Mr. Ryerson would be forced to make other arrangements for physician coverage at the Jackson/Bagley health center.

The Charlotte health center was staffed on a part-time basis (20 hours a week) by Dr. Christina Calder, an arrangement also made by Dr. White. Dr. White originally had recruited internist Calder for the MHMG, but her membership had been blocked by the group's internist on the basis that another internist would not be a good addition. At that point, which was the summer of 1976, Dr. White persuaded Dr. Calder to practice at the Charlotte health center, and her desire to practice only part-time met with the approval of the Palowee River Regional Health Services. Dr. Calder therefore represented the only physician provider available to Mr. Ryerson outside the MHMG. He did not want to jeopardize that resource but somehow had to expand physician coverage at the health center, and the only possibility for the near future was by utilizing the MHMG.*

Next Steps

By the end of August 1977, Mr. Ryerson had completed the first phase of his job: gathering information. He felt that he now was ready to identify the steps needed to accomplish his goal of developing two successful primary care health centers and mobilizing a regional board. In addition to the complexities surrounding that goal, Mr. Ryerson also had another complication to contend with: his growing involvement in hospital matters beyond the scope of his job.

Earlier in the month, Mr. Ryerson had met with Dr. Calder to discuss her role and her feelings about the project. Although Dr. White had described how Dr. Calder became associated with the Charlotte center, Mr. Ryerson wanted to find out first-hand whether she would be receptive to him as the new health center administrator and to the possibility of working with MHMG physicians. During the meeting, Dr. Calder had been cautious in expressing her opinions, especially about the MHMG. Nonetheless, Mr. Ryerson was satisfied that he had established the foundation for a good working relationship and, as a result, was over one hurdle. His satisfaction stemmed from

---

*As of August 1977, the Morgan Hill Medical Group consisted of three physicians in addition to general practitioner White: a surgeon, an obstetric/gynecologic practitioner and an internist, the latter two being foreign medical graduates.

Dr. Calder's acceptance of the position of part-time medical director at Charlotte in return for agreeing to consider working with any qualified physicians Mr. Ryerson could recruit, including the MHMG physicians if needed.

Another step that Mr. Ryerson had recently taken was the hiring of the public accounting firm of Ernst & Whinney to conduct a financial and administrative analysis of the two health centers. Mr. Ryerson thought that the use of "outside experts" to evaluate the health centers and present the findings would appear less intimidating to the health center staffs and the community groups than if presented by Ryerson himself.

Mr. Ryerson would be confronting his greatest obstacles, however, in the following week, when he had several meetings scheduled. He was to meet individually with the Palowee River Regional Health Services, the Jackson Area Health Services and the Jackson Improvement Association and wanted to be ready with a plan that somehow would integrate the diverse interests and concerns of those community groups with his own needs in establishing the primary care regional network. Mr. Ryerson viewed it as somewhat of a coup that the groups, and particularly the JIA, had even agreed to meet with him. He had used Dr. White's influence and contacts to set up the meetings.

Mr. Ryerson also had a meeting scheduled with Roger Hawley. Although its main purpose was to brief Mr. Hawley on his progress and to outline his approach in terms of how the hospital fit in, Mr. Ryerson also wanted to broach the subject of his role at the hospital, which recently seemed to be taking on new meaning.

Exhibit Objectives for Health Centers*

---

1. To provide comprehensive primary care to the medically underserved population of 25,411 in northern Greene County in Maine through satellite centers located in the villages of Charlotte and Jackson/Bagley supported by the staff and facilities of C.T. Meyer Hospital of Morgan Hill.

2. To create a practice structure that supplements and extends the ability of the present physicians to provide quality primary care in this area, to include optimum utilization of ancillary personnel, and that allows the C.T. Meyer Hospital of Morgan Hill to realize its potential for service to its area constituents by the creation of a hospital-laboratory-specialist available milieu that will attract physicians both to come and to remain.

3. To qualify this effort for family practice residency training.

4. To intimately involve the service recipients in this device for care.

5. To establish a financially feasible program that will meet the near optimum medical needs of the area.

6. Through critical analysis, to assist the community in determining future levels of professional care required for its health needs.

---

*Submitted by C.T. Meyer Hospital of Morgan Hill in Innovations in Ambulatory Primary Care grant application, 1976.

7
University Medical Center

University Medical Center

In July 1978, Cole Latimar was hired by University Medical Center (UMC) as administrator for a primary care center that was to open soon in the rural Green Grove Valley area in northern California. The Suncook Family Health Center (Suncook) facility was owned by the nonprofit community corporation, Suncook Development, but was operated as an outpatient satellite of UMC.

The new health center, which opened in September 1978, was met with open arms by the medically underserved population of the 30-square-mile service area, and utilization increased rapidly. The center was located in temporary quarters in the town of Greenville until construction of a new facility was completed. Physician resources were plentiful because of Suncook's affiliation with UMC, a teaching facility.

Suncook had been open for more than one and one-half years when UMC first became aware of a sizable billing backlog at Suncook, according to Dr. Cranston Parsons, assistant professor of medicine and chief of the section of general internal medicine, who also was the UMC's director for the Suncook project. Dr. Parsons reported the following:

> Apparently, Suncook began experiencing a billing backlog not long after opening because by the time we [UMC] heard about it, there was more than $50,000 in patient charges that hadn't even been billed to patients or insurers. Obviously, the problem had to be building for some time to have reached that point. UMC had no inkling of the situation because of Cole Latimar's method of reporting. On his monthly reports, which were our only way of getting information on Suncook's activity, Mr. Latimar wasn't reporting the actual collection rate. Instead, he was using the monthly collection rate of UMC's outpatient department to estimate Suncook's collections in his reports. We had no knowledge of the severity of the collection problem at Suncook until the spring of 1980, when Mr. Latimar came to us for approval to

hire more billers to reduce the billing backlog. I guess he figured he could handle it or that the problem wasn't all that acute. Cash flow wasn't a problem for Suncook because UMC was providing whatever operating funds were needed above the revenue they were taking in.

Cole Latimar had a different version of the situation:

I certainly wasn't hiding anything from UMC. The problem was the double-billing system we were using at Suncook—it was so complex and so tied into UMC's billing methods that it was nearly impossible for me to have an accurate picture of anything at any given time. It was UMC's decision that Suncook use the system in the first place. At the time, that decision sounded logical to me because it coincided with our objective of maximizing third-party reimbursement for our patient charges and we fully expected to bill manually on a temporary basis until hooking into UMC's automated billing system. That just never happened, though, because UMC was having its own computer start-up delays.

Another factor, as I look back, was that I started out doing the billing myself and continued it for four months, rather than hiring a biller from the start, which was, once again, UMC's decision. Things just mushroomed from there, but I couldn't get UMC's people concerned. I brought the matter up to Dr. Parsons on several occasions, and I'm sure Dr. Endicott, Suncook's medical director, reported the situation to his superiors at UMC, too. I guess it finally sank in when the figure exceeded $50,000 and there were several months worth of uncollected receivables. I was making sure that we took care of the most urgent bills—those we sent in for Medi-Cal reimbursement, which had a 90-day limit after the date of service to be eligible. We were meeting that deadline so we weren't losing any Medi-Cal revenue. We weren't actually losing any revenue because of the backlog, but I knew that the longer the bills were delayed, the more difficult it would be to collect from patients.

UMC's Charter

University Medical Center is a campus of the state university system, encompassing a state-supported medical school and a teaching hospital that opened in 1976 with 100 of its planned 400 beds. The school had a dual charter: to emphasize the training of primary care physicians and to improve access to primary medical care for the medically underserved citizens of the northern quarter of the state. The UMC had to become a recognized tertiary care center in order to attract faculty, and it needed practice sites for its residents in family practice, internal medicine and pediatrics. The hospital therefore was planned as an ultimate referral facility for an integrated health care network of primary care centers and community hospitals throughout the northern portion of the state.

Until Suncook opened in September 1978, however, the extent of UMC's involvement in primary care delivery in underserved areas consisted of the Family Practice Department's affiliation with one urban and two rural primary care centers owned and operated by independent community corporations. UMC's Family Practice Department had arranged with those corporations to place residents in their facilities.

Formation of Suncook Family Health Center

In 1975, a group of concerned Greenville citizens approached UMC for help in attracting physicians to the Green Grove Valley area. They met with Wendell Jones, M.D., associate dean for primary care, who authorized a university study that verified a severe physician shortage in Green Grove Valley. Dr. Jones concluded that the needs of the area's population for medical care and of UMC for practice sites could be met simultaneously by establishing a primary care center.

Dr. Jones' plan was to set up a model internal medicine/pediatrics site. Recognizing that they lacked a primary care training site for their residents, the chairmen of the two UMC clinical departments were very receptive to the idea of setting up a model program in Greenville to serve Green Grove Valley.

Dr. Jones appointed Dr. Parsons to serve as UMC's director for the Greenville project. It was Dr. Parsons' job to formalize arrangements with the Greenville community group, which was organizing into the Suncook Development Corporation, as well as to seek funds for the primary care center, to set up the facility and to serve as UMC's project director for the center once it was operational.

Under the arrangement between the university and Suncook Development Corporation, the corporation was the owner of the Greenville facility and responsible for supervising construction and for future maintenance; the university leased the building from the corporation. Besides being the landlord, the Suncook Development Corporation was an advisory board to UMC for the center. The two organizations collaborated to raise start-up funds (from grants and community sources*), and UMC was responsible for subsidizing the center's ongoing operations until it reached self-sufficiency (projected to occur after four years), at which point UMC would provide only a $40,000 annual stipend to cover the cost of physician preceptorship for its residents at Suncook.

The link with UMC provided both direct and indirect benefits for Suncook: physician recruitment, rotating residents, compensation, fringe benefits, clinical services beyond the center's capabilities and administrative support services such as purchasing and accounting.

The Suncook center also established a formal relationship with the local Chico-Redding Regional Hospital—a secondary care community hospital with a 135-bed main facility in Chico and a subdivision in Redding—that benefited all parties concerned. Suncook's physicians could admit their local patients there, which in turn alleviated concern by the local hospital and its medical staff that they would lose inpatients to UMC. The UMC benefited by gaining a secondary care training site and referral base without risking accusations of setting up Suncook to fill its own beds. Among the benefits it afforded Suncook were a local resource for hospitalizing patients and a stimulant for recruiting physicians.

Organizational Ties between Suncook and UMC

The Suncook Family Health Center operated similarly to a group practice, with Mr. Latimar as administrator/group practice manager reporting to Dr. Glen Endicott, the medical director. Both men had been recruited by UMC for the Suncook project. Mr. Latimar's previous experience, after earning an M.B.A. with a health care

---

*Grants were awarded by the Hospital Research and Educational Trust ($76,000 for one year) and the federal Health Underserved Rural Areas program ($200,000 for 1977 and $150,000 for 1978). Community contributions included $65,000 from community members, the donation of land for the permanent facility and $20,000 from the Chico-Redding Regional Hospital.

emphasis in 1975, was as a manager in the ambulatory care division of a large metropolitan hospital in California. Medical director Endicott had completed his residency in pediatrics in Ohio and practiced in Colorado for 18 years before joining Suncook. Both men reported that they enjoyed a good working relationship and seldom encountered any problem of overlapping responsibilities. Beyond that point, however, the organizational ties to UMC were complex and were made even more so by extrinsic relationships that evolved over time.

According to the organizational chart *(Figure 1),* Dr. Endicott was accountable to the chairmen of UMC's Internal Medicine and Pediatrics Departments, to Mark Steinberg, a UMC administrator, and to the Suncook Development Corporation. However, Dr. Endicott's accountabilities to the two clinical departments and his responsibilities as a full-time Suncook provider, a preceptor for the residents who rotated there and medical director left him little opportunity to interact with Mr. Steinberg, despite the formal organizational structure. As a result, Mr. Latimar was the health center's primary liaison with Mr. Steinberg. Mr. Latimar's interaction with Mr. Steinberg, however, was limited because of a reporting relationship that did not even appear on the organizational chart but nonetheless represented the closest link between the two organizations: the relationship involving Dr. Parsons, UMC's project director for Suncook. Initially, Dr. Parsons had planned to take the post of medical director at Suncook as well, but had decided against that approach and hired Dr. Endicott in order to avoid a full-time commitment at Suncook. In addition to maintaining direct communication with Suncook through Mr. Latimar, Dr. Parsons often·involved UMC's part-time director of ambulatory care, Roberta Buxton, in the Suncook project.

Mr. Latimar had the following to say about his organizational relationships with UMC:

> One structure was defined on paper, but another was actually in effect. Because of Dr. Endicott's clinical responsibilities, I was the link to UMC, at least for the nonmedical issues. It wasn't that simple, though, because I was never sure who to go to at UMC—Mr. Steinberg, Dr. Parsons or Miss Buxton. When I tried to follow the defined path by going to Mr. Steinberg, Dr. Parsons would resent it. On the other hand, Dr. Parsons either didn't have the connections to resolve my problems or he chose not to use them. Dr. Parsons and Miss Buxton had done a good job in the planning stages but now there were operational issues facing us. I think Dr. Parsons and Miss Buxton

Figure 1 Organizational Structure of University Medical Center/Suncook Family Health Center

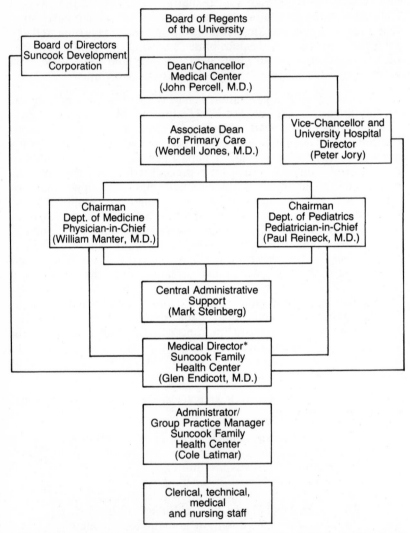

* The medical director, appointed by the dean/chancellor of the university and approved by the Suncook Development Corporation board of directors, reports to the chairpersons of the respective medical school departments for professional and educational activities, to the vice-chancellor and university hospital director for administrative activities, and to the Suncook board of directors for approval of general policy issues.

viewed Suncook as their baby and didn't want to loosen their hold by giving me some administrative freedom or by involving others at UMC. Dr. Parsons was interested in Suncook more from a policy or control standpoint. For example, he wanted to maintain all contacts with grant agencies; I had to refer all questions from grantors to him. Dr. Parsons was sincere about wanting Suncook to succeed but he was a doctor, not an administrator.

Actually, Mr. Steinberg was the most help to me. He was head of central administrative support at UMC, so he could relate better to my needs and had the ties to the UMC administrative support systems to address them. I would go to him for help in untangling the mess Suncook always ran into with the shared purchasing arrangement, and he had the contacts and know-how to at least expedite matters. Mr. Steinberg recognized that the reporting requirements to the two grant agencies were an added burden on me and did everything he could to lighten that load. He also took a big interest in the negotiations that were going on with the computer supplier to hook Suncook up to the billing system at UMC. That wasn't his direct responsibility, but he understood our situation and wanted to help if he could.

As far as Dr. Parsons was concerned, the problem was not the complex organizational structure between UMC and Suncook but Mr. Latimar's reluctance to take direction from him. Dr. Parsons stated: "The organizational structure would have been easy enough to deal with if Mr. Latimar had been receptive to my role and Miss Buxton's. There were many instances when we showed him a way to resolve a particular problem, but he ignored us."

Mr. Latimar viewed the ties to UMC with mixed feelings. On the positive side, Suncook had a built-in physician supply, a guaranteed influx of operating funds until becoming self-sustaining and a savings in both time and expense by relying on UMC's personnel and financial systems. Some of those advantages, however, proved to be a burden to Suncook, as Mr. Latimar illustrated:

Under the shared purchasing arrangement, I did the paperwork [purchase order] and sent it to UMC, which ordered the item from the vendor. After the item was delivered to Suncook, the vendor naturally expected payment. However, the university was responsible for issuing payment and it typically took them six months to do so. Meanwhile, because my name was on the purchase order and the item was delivered here, the vendor would be breathing down my neck for payment.

In July of 1979, we decided to apply to the Farmers Home Administration for a loan to refinance the center's mortgage, which would save us $700 a month. The Suncook board, which was the mortgage holder, agreed with the plan and so did Dr. Parsons. However, the Farmers Home Administration required a 20-year lease guarantee to approve the refinancing, and UMC was lessee, which meant a policy-level decision by the university. I therefore had to present the refinancing idea to the university and work through its legal staff to hammer out the negotiations between the three parties—the Suncook board, the university and the lending institution. We got the mortgage refinanced, but it took 14 months.

It was the billing system at Suncook, however, that proved to be Mr. Latimar's biggest problem and, to him, the most glaring illustration of the UMC bureaucracy.

UMC's Billing System

Suncook used the same double-billing system that UMC used, which generated two bills (or claim forms) for each patient visit—one for the facility component and one for the professional component of the charge. UMC segregated its billing system in order to provide a separate account for the group practice comprising its medical faculty. UMC had formed this group practice structure for the medical faculty in order to augment the regular faculty salary paid by the university, which was inadequate to attract medical staff as faculty members and to compensate them for their patient care services. All income from professional charges was applied to the group practice account to accommodate this salary differential.

UMC elected the group practice structure—and hence the double-billing system—to compensate its medical faculty rather than contracting with the physicians for professional services rendered. A contract would have to be brought before the university board of regents and the state legislature, an approach the medical center wished to avoid.

Suncook's Billing System

Because Suncook was in a rural service area where the median family income was $9,600, the health center needed a billing system that would maximize third-party reimbursement and minimize out-of-pocket expense to the patient. Preliminary estimates of the payer class distribution of Suncook's patients were 40 percent for Blue Cross/Blue Shield and 15 percent each for Medi-Cal, Medicare, commercial insurers and self-pay.

Before Suncook opened, UMC's external consultant conducted a study on billing alternatives for the health center. The study showed that, depending on how the health center was classified, it could expect to collect from 60 to 88 percent of its charges from all reimbursement sources *(Figure 2)*. Based on this study, Dr. Parsons selected the alternative that classified Suncook as a hospital outpatient department staffed by private physicians. Potentially, this alternative would allow Suncook to collect 75 percent of its charges to all insurers, the second highest collection rate of the classifications presented by the consultant. The alternative with the highest collection rate (that is, a hospital outpatient department staffed by hospital-employed physicians) was not feasible because of the physician group practice structure at UMC.

Given this classification selection and Dr. Parsons' rejection of a separate automated billing system at Suncook based on the price quoted by UMC's computer supplier, the consultant recommended that Suncook use the same billing system as UMC and link up to it via a computer terminal.

As is typical in an ambulatory care setting, Suncook generated a high volume of low-unit charges. The activities a biller performed related to a relatively small amount of revenue; for example, a biller may spend 10 minutes processing a $15 charge for a 10-minute patient visit.

Suncook operated the billing system manually *(Figure 3)*. For each patient visit eligible for third-party coverage (estimated at 85 percent of Suncook's business), Suncook generated two claim forms—one for the facility and one for the professional component. The forms were sent directly to the third-party payers. Payment was made either to Suncook or to UMC, depending on the third-party payer and whether it was a facility or a professional charge *(Figure 4)*. For payments made directly to UMC, Suncook had to await receipt of the remittance verification from UMC before it could bill the patient for any disallowed charges.

Figure 2 Suncook Family Health Center Classifications and Billing Systems Options

Classification	Single/Double Bill Implication	Third-Party Payer Implications			% Estimated Bad Debt and Contractual Adjustments
		Blue Cross/Blue Shield	Medicare Parts A and B	Medi-Cal Hospital/Physician Programs	
Private practice	Single	Charges submitted to Blue Shield. Payment based on restrictive profiles. Physician visits not a reimbursable service.	Charges submitted to Part B. Payment based on restrictive profiles.	Charges submitted to Medi-Cal physician program, which pays on a fixed-fee basis. Fees would recognize less than 50% of costs.	40
Neighborhood health center	Single	Same as above	Same as above	Charges submitted to Medi-Cal hospital program, which takes cost into consideration. However, would require time-consuming cost reporting.	35
Hospital OPD staffed by private physicians	Double	Charges submitted to Blue Shield for physician services and Blue Cross for facility-related charges. Blue Cross considers OPD visits to be a reimbursable charge. Blue Cross payment based on costs.	Charges submitted to Part B for physician services and Part A for facility-related charges. Part A payment based on costs.	Charges submitted to Medi-Cal physician program for physician services and Medi-Cal hospital program for facility charges. Medi-Cal hospital program payment based on costs.	25
Hospital OPD staffed by hospital-employed physicians	Single	All charges submitted to Blue Cross. Payment based on costs.	All charges submitted to Medicare Part A. Payment based on costs.	All charges submitted to Medi-Cal hospital program. Payment based on costs.	12

Reflecting on the decision to use UMC's billing system, Mr. Latimar stated: "At the time, it made sense to me because of the reimbursement advantage it gave Suncook. We were already tied into UMC and I figured it would help me out if they performed some of the billing steps for us. Also, we fully expected to link up to their computer system, so the portion we had to do at Suncook would be automated as well."

Figure 3 Billing Process of Suncook Family Health Center

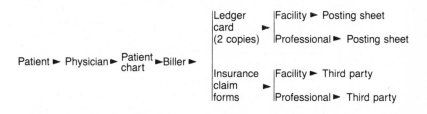

Figure 4 Reimbursement Process of Suncook (SK) Family Health Center

Facility Payment

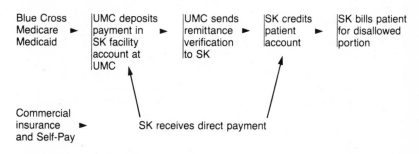

Professional Payment

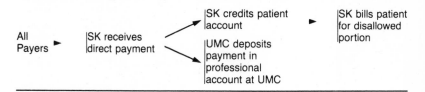

Mr. Latimar performed the billing for Suncook when it first opened because, as he stated, "Dr. Parsons directed me to, and since we were just starting up, I didn't believe it would be enough of a burden on me to make a case about it. Our original plan of having one biller for every two physicians was never implemented at the outset and later became totally unrealistic." Mr. Latimar soon became inundated with the billing work load and convinced UMC that he needed to hire a biller. Marcia Rubin started in January 1979 after training several weeks at the UMC Billing Department. At the time Miss Rubin was hired, Suncook had three full-time physicians.

The addition of billing clerk Rubin did little to improve the situation. In the months of May and June 1979, charges totaled $18,713 compared with collections of $1,696. Mr. Latimar received UMC's approval to add a temporary biller. The temporary biller worked for three months and the result was reflected in the collections for August. The improvement was short-lived, however, as the collection rate fell in the subsequent months. Mr. Latimar attributed that to the hiring of a new permanent biller who was being trained by Miss Rubin, resulting in lower overall productivity during the training period. Mr. Latimar again sought the university's help, this time for UMC billers who could be borrowed by Suncook on a temporary basis. By June 1980, Suncook had a complement of eight billers and $78,132 in charges for which no bills had been generated *(Figures 5 and 6).*

Mr. Latimar blamed the situation on the billing system itself:

> It was complicated to begin with because it generated two bills for each visit. UMC may have been able to handle the complexity of a double-billing system because it had an up-and-running billing department and, despite some recurring computer billing problems, was nearly automated. We didn't have those luxuries at Suncook.

Figure 5 Suncook Family Health Center Billing Backlog Chronology–9/1/78-6/30/80

Time period	Charges this period	Billed charges this period	Unbilled charges this period	Total unbilled charges*
9/1/78–12/13/78	$ 18,791	$ 13,644	$ 5,146	$ 5,146
1/1/79–06/30/79	38,284	28,729	9,554	14,701
7/1/79–12/31/79	85,393	50,594	34,798	49,499
1/1/80–06/30/80	154,537	125,904	28,632	78,132

*Cumulative figures.

What we did have at Suncook was added complexities. First, we had a manual operation. Second, we had timing delays because we had to wait for the remittance verifications from UMC before billing patients for disallowed charges. And third, it was almost impossible for me, or for anyone, to have an accurate record of receivables. Payments actually came to both places, but because UMC maintained the accounts, they had the records, not us. However, they had only the payment records and not the billing information, so there was little relationship between the two when the billings got behind. We both used the same provider numbers for third-party claims, although Suncook's were prefixed with "SK." The problem was that the prefix sometimes got dropped in the process, so the payment couldn't be associated with a Suncook service. That botched up the receivables, as well as our own individual patient accounts.

Figure 6 Suncook Family Health Center Utilization by Month, 9/1/78-6/30/80

	Month	Patient Visits
1978	September	76
	October	224
	November	195
	December	254
1979	January	288
	February	306
	March	311
	April	310
	May	440
	June	534
	July	499
	August	663
	September	535
	October	747
	November	1,055
	December	801
1980	January	1,204
	February	1,159
	March	1,192
	April	1,260
	May	1,301
	June	1,110

The billing procedure was pretty confusing to patients, too. For one visit to Suncook, John Doe might
receive a facility component bill and a professional
component bill payable to Suncook, plus benefit
summary forms from Blue Cross and Blue Shield. He
might get those two bills for one visit at different
times depending on when and if Suncook received the
remittance verification from UMC. If he had an
inquiry, he probably wouldn't know whether to call
us or UMC.

Mr. Latimar's concern with the billing backlog was not one of cash
flow because the medical center covered the outstanding charges;
rather, it was one of credibility. Because the Suncook Family Health
Center intended to become self-sufficient, Mr. Latimar believed the
billing backlog represented a credibility barrier in convincing the
medical center of Suncook's ability to achieve that objective. He also
saw a potential credibility problem with the Suncook service area:
"People are probably wondering where their bills are, are probably
having difficulty budgeting for their visits and may not even remember
having been here for a visit."

Roberta Buxton was not very sympathetic to Mr. Latimar's plight
because she and Dr. Parsons had offered him a solution that he never
acted on. Miss Buxton said, "When we began realizing the extent of
the problem, which was after Mr. Latimar borrowed some of the
UMC billers but still couldn't reverse the backlog, we offered him a
way out. We suggested that Suncook merely send its patient encounter
forms directly to UMC, and we would do the billing from there. It
would have simplified things tremendously for Suncook. We never
heard from Mr. Latimar that he would accept the plan."

Mr. Latimar explained his rejection of that idea as follows:
"Frankly, I didn't want to give UMC any more control over Suncook's
operations. It might have solved the immediate problem of billing but
would have exacerbated the big picture in the long run, especially
since I knew Suncook would have to be self-sufficient. I thought that
we should identify other options and evaluate them, not just act
hastily on what Dr. Parsons or Miss Buxton wanted. Another factor
was my belief that we would be more responsive to patient inquiries
than UMC could be."

Time Is Running Out

By September 1980, Mr. Latimar saw that his stop-gap measure of
hiring or borrowing more and more billers was not working, nor had

any consensus been reached on the promised automation of Suncook's billing procedures. He felt that the seriousness of the situation had finally been recognized by UMC, but he was unsure of what steps would be taken to address it. It was now two years since Suncook had opened, and UMC was planning to conduct an evaluation of the health center in November to determine whether it should continue supporting Suncook and, if so, to what extent.

Mr. Latimar knew that UMC had a big investment in Suncook, not only in terms of the two years of financial support already expended, but also as a future practice site for its residency programs. UMC was already making plans to double the number of residents assigned to Suncook from four to eight. He also knew that several people at UMC had a stake in Suncook and wanted it to succeed—Dr. Parsons, Mr. Steinberg and the two clinical department heads among others. Also, the medical center's credibility as a training site for future primary care physicians hinged, to some extent, on Suncook's success.

Mr. Latimar wondered whether he should let UMC work out the problems with the billing system or whether he should come up with his own plan for resolving them. If he elected the latter course, he wondered what options he could consider that would work and that could show promise of results in time for the November evaluation.

8
Hemming ford

Hemmingford

Three years after the Community Medical Center of Northwest Delaware County, Ohio, had been awarded a grant from the Hospital Research and Educational Trust for start-up funding, it was one of the most successful of the two dozen primary care centers funded under the demonstration project. Its success during those three years could be measured in a number of areas: commitments of over one million dollars from government and private sources and an additional $150,000 from the community; the ease of physician and other professional staff recruitment; a full patient load; a newly built, modern facility; a strong community board that worked closely with the health center administrator; the establishment of supportive relationships with other area health providers; and the addition of dental services to a comprehensive range of primary medical services.

Despite these accomplishments, however, the Community Medical Center's administrator was concerned about several pressing problems facing the center at the start of its fourth year of operation, not the least of which was achieving financial solvency.

Northwest Delaware County

Northwest Delaware County is a rural Appalachian mountain region a few miles from the West Virginia panhandle *(Figure 1)*. Its 12 political subdivisions cover approximately 240 square miles. Centrally located Hemmingford, with a population of 2,118, is approximately 35 miles from Pittsburgh. At the 1970 census, 29 percent of the region's population was under 15 years of age, 10 percent was above 65, the mean annual income was $8,153 and 9.6 percent of the families were below the poverty level. The economy is dependent on agriculture, titanium mining and processing, steel processing and construction.

In 1973, northwestern Delaware County had only six physicians for its 25,000 residents. All were general practitioners and three were reaching retirement age. The physician-to-population ratio of 1:4,160 was one-seventh the national average. There were only seven full-time dentists practicing in the area, placing the dentist-to-population ratio just slightly above the physician-to-population ratio. Residents needing medical attention typically faced long waits for appointments or traveled from 30 to 60 minutes to the nearest hospital emergency room for treatment.

Figure 1 Delaware County, Ohio

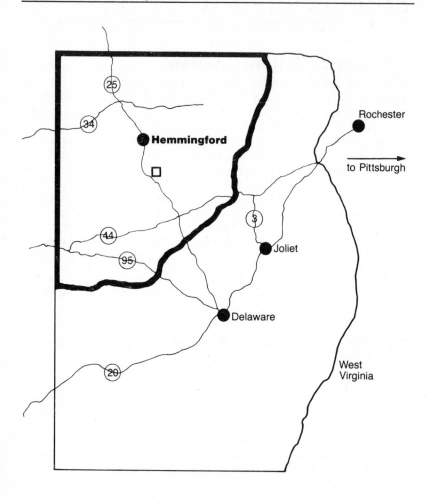

Hemmingford

Rochester

to Pittsburgh

3

Joliet

Delaware

West
Virginia

25

34

44

95

20

Key

 25 Highways
● Towns
▬ Health center service area
□ Permanent health center location

The hospital closest to Hemmingford was Joliet General, 12 miles away, with 105 acute care beds and an emergency room. Fifteen miles in another direction was Delaware Hospital, with 484 acute care beds, an emergency room and an organized outpatient department.

Community Initiates Action

In 1972, Local 1311 of the United Auto Workers, representing 180 employees of the Activated Titanium Company located just outside Hemmingford, decided to initiate attempts to expand the primary care resources in northwest Delaware County. The local union's president appointed a four-member committee to tackle that goal. Bill Marshall, a past vice-president of the local who had lived and worked in the region most of his 48 years, was a natural choice to head the committee. The initial efforts of Local 1311, and particularly Bill Marshall, laid the groundwork for the comprehensive ambulatory primary care center that opened in July 1976.

Under the leadership of husky Bill Marshall, a well-known community organizer who dabbled in local politics, the union committee that was organized in 1972 set out to involve as many community members as possible in its task of finding medical resources for the region. By holding meetings around the area, the group identified several other residents who had an interest in the project and were willing to devote their time to it. Among them were two registered nurses and several people who served as volunteers for health and social welfare organizations.

A Corporation Forms

In February 1973, the community group formed a private, non-profit corporation—Community Medical Center (CMC) of Northwest Delaware County, Inc.—to seek funds for a primary care health center. The corporation consisted of one representative from each of the 12 political subdivisions comprising the proposed service area for the center. The corporation adopted bylaws, elected Mr. Marshall as president and appointed executive, finance, personnel recruiting, nominating, location and government committees. As time passed and new needs emerged, the committees were restructured (for example, in late 1975, the location committee became the building and grounds committee and supervised facility construction).

During the next three years of biweekly meetings, the CMC corporation made several advances toward its goal. First, the CMC received 501(c)(3) tax status. Second, the CMC conducted a survey to identify local health needs and assess the potential community contribution base. The survey indicated that obtaining medical care was a problem for nearly half the residents of the 240-square-mile area and that contributions could be expected from the community despite its economic characteristics. Third, the corporation secured federal designation of the region as a health manpower shortage area, opening the door to federal and other funding sources. Finally, staff of the local Comprehensive Health Planning Agency, the forerunner of the Health Systems Agency, worked with the corporation in planning and organizing its efforts. Later, the Health Systems Agency formally endorsed all aspects of the project, including programs and facility.

The successes of the community group, although noteworthy, meant little without financial resources to start a health center. Raising money therefore was the corporation's major challenge. The CMC wanted to raise $100,000 in capital development funds during 1975. Undaunted by the magnitude of this goal given the economic status of the population, Mr. Marshall applied his characteristic zeal and tenacity to lead the CMC in what a local newspaper called "the most ambitious fund drive that this part of Appalachia has ever seen."

Mr. Marshall knew that the corporation would need practical help from an experienced fund raiser. He turned to Dave Youngberg, who was the executive director and a successful fund raiser for the Pittsburgh chapter of the American Cancer Society. The two had met several years earlier when working for the Boy Scouts of America, Mr. Youngberg as an employee and Mr. Marshall as a volunteer. The CMC president convinced Mr. Youngberg to volunteer his help in conducting the local fund drive. With Mr. Youngberg's assistance, the CMC recruited 500 volunteer fund raisers from the community, and the campaign exceeded its goal. Community residents pledged $100,000 and local businesses and religious organizations pledged another $44,000.

An Administrator Is Hired

Mr. Marshall and the other CMC members were impressed with Mr. Youngberg. As Mr. Marshall stated it: "He comes off as being pretty soft-spoken and easy-going—not the type you would think of as a dynamo fund raiser and a go-getter. But underneath, that's just what he was. He had a lot of skill in organizing and in relating to people, as he proved to us in our fund drive. He's a very likable fellow. He also had a lot of concern and interest in our project. He wasn't even a member of our community but worked as hard as anyone here did."

The CMC board offered Mr. Youngberg the job of administrator for the medical center, feeling that his experience in administration and fund raising for nonprofit organizations more than offset his limited health care background. Mr. Youngberg accepted the offer and assumed his new post in March 1976.

The CMC's new administrator pursued every possible avenue to funding for the center, including foundation and government grant sources. His efforts produced $1,078,760 for the first three years of operation: $110,000 in federal Hill-Burton construction funds; $75,000 from the Kresge Foundation for construction; $23,500 for planning and $100,000 for first-year operations from the Ohio Department of Health; $75,000 from small private foundations; $84,500 from the Appalachian Regional Commission for equipment, which was awarded jointly with a federal Rural Health Initiative grant of $199,760 for start-up and first-year operations*; an additional commitment of $120,000 each for years two and three of operations from the Rural Health Initiative program; $141,000 from the Hospital Research and Educational Trust for two years; and $30,000 for a National Health Service Corps nurse practitioner for two years.

Progress toward opening the center was being made in other arenas as well. With help from Joliet General Hospital, the CMC recruited Dr. Wa San Lee, who had just completed two years of postgraduate work at Cook County (IL) Hospital. The CMC also recruited a registered nurse and a receptionist/bookkeeper. Along with fund raising and recruitment, Mr. Youngberg was traveling to other primary care centers in the state to learn all he could about their operations. The 32-year-old administrator was by this time an active and informed member of his new community, familiar with and sensitive to its political nuances and a volunteer worker for local social welfare organizations.

The Medical Center Opens

The CMC located a building in the center of Hemmingford to house the center until a permanent facility could be constructed. The temporary storefront quarters were remodeled, and in July 1976, after more than four years of hard work by the CMC, the center opened its doors with a staff of four. In the first month, Dr. Lee treated 152 patients. Two months later, Betty Ramsey, a nurse practitioner assignee from the National Health Service Corps, began at the center.

---

*As an illustration of the work required to obtain funding, the CMC's combined application to the Appalachian Regional Commission and the Rural Health Initiative program comprised approximately 300 pages.

Accomplishing Objectives

In a grant application filed by the CMC in August 1976, the corporation projected serving 5,840 patients, for a total of 7,008 patient visits, in its first full calendar-year of operation. The application also listed seven broad objectives for the health center as well as specific objectives to be accomplished in each of the first two full years of operation.

After six months of operation, the Community Medical Center was making good progress toward accomplishing its objectives. A total of 1,162 patients—an average of 194 per month—had used the center. Health education pamphlets were printed and distributed to patients, and the center and its services were publicized in local newspapers. Services already offered included routine medical treatment, child immunizations, minor emergency care, basic lab tests, medical histories on new patients, self-help and prevention, plus periodic immunization, screening, mental health and WIC programs conducted at the center in cooperation with state and county health offices.

Mr. Youngberg began interviewing a second physician candidate as early as November 1976. Working relationships had been established with area hospitals to gain support for the center and contacts initiated with area physicians in an attempt to alleviate potential apprehension about the center competing with their practices. Several members of the CMC had received appointments to the governing board of Joliet General Hospital. A target date of October 1977 had been set to occupy a permanent facility, and plans for its construction were under way.

The CMC board's evolution from an organizer and fund raiser into a policymaking body was proceeding smoothly according to administrator Youngberg. Bill Marshall continued to be the driving force behind the board and stopped by the center each day to see how things were going. Although Mr. Youngberg and Mr. Marshall occasionally had differences of opinion, they seemed able to resolve disagreements. Mr. Youngberg's pragmatism and Mr. Marshall's grandiose visions seemed to balance each other to produce a hard-working team effort for the CMC.

Physician Resources

In July 1977, the board signed an initial one-year contract with Patrick Kolb, M.D., a recent graduate of Delaware Hospital's family practice residency program, to become the center's second physician. Before summer ended, Dr. Kolb had indicated his willingness to renew for three additional years (Dr. Lee had already renewed for three years in January 1977).

With the addition of a second physician, the CMC anticipated that patient utilization would double from approximately 200 to 400 new patients a month. But center growth was not the only reason for adding a second physician. Both Mr. Youngberg and the board saw the addition as providing other important benefits, such as a reduction in Dr. Lee's work load and better after-hours coverage arrangements.

Having gained a second physician, the board wanted to provide 24-hour physician coverage at the center. Mr. Youngberg convinced them this was not financially feasible because the physicians were paid based on the number of hours worked. Instead, center hours were expanded in July from 40 to 60 per week, the volunteer answering service for emergencies was continued and the two physicians alternated on-call coverage weekly.

Dr. Lee had staff privileges at both Joliet and Delaware hospitals, but tended to refer patients almost exclusively to Delaware Hospital because it had better facilities and convenient highway access. (Joliet Hospital was attempting to obtain Health Systems Agency approval to rebuild its obsolete facility.) Dr. Kolb elected to secure staff privileges at Delaware Hospital, where he had completed his residency.

The physicians' contracts required that they spend a minimum of 40 hours each week providing care at the center, including a specified minimum number of evening and Saturday hours, for which they received a set salary *(see Exhibit)*. Time spent in treating patients in the hospital—typically 5 to 10 hours a week each—was not covered by the contract, and revenues generated by those visits accrued directly to the physicians. Mr. Youngberg estimated that each CMC physician generated an additional $10,000 to $15,000 annually from treating center patients who were hospitalized.

Mr. Youngberg explained the rationale for this type of physician contract: "When I visited other clinics that were similar to the CMC, I found that where the contract didn't set a requirement on the number of hours at the center, the physicians were spending extra time at the hospital and cutting back their time at the clinic. I wanted to make sure our physicians spent at least 40 hours at the center so that we would meet the federal standard of a minimum of 4,200 encounters per year."

By the end of 1977, the center had been operating for six months with two physicians. The CMC's projected increase in new patient volume based on the addition of Dr. Kolb had not materialized

(Figure 2). Confused by this discrepancy, Mr. Youngberg could think of only one factor to explain it—one area physician expected to retire had continued practicing.

1977 Financial Picture

Patient charges for the services provided at CMC were set by the board based on the type of service and the provider. The fees charged for physician services were competitive with area physicians and based on the length of time spent with the patient—$5 for a *brief* visit of 7½ minutes or less, $10 for a *basic* visit (the most prevalent type of patient visit at the center) and $15 for an *extended* visit of more than 15 minutes. Separate fees were set for follow-up nurse care ($4 per encounter), medication and ancillary services. The physicians were responsible for identifying the type of visit (brief, basic or extended) on the patient's chart for billing purposes. Mr. Youngberg reported that the physicians, particularly Dr. Kolb, were reluctant to charge the extended visit rate and often charged the brief visit rate for basic visits.

The center's average charge for a patient visit during 1977 was $10.99, for which the cost to the center averaged $24.22. Gross revenue from patients and third parties was slightly above $78,000,

Figure 2 Medical Care* Utilization by Month 7/76-6/79

	New Patients†				Patient Visits			
	1976‡	1977	1978	1979	1976	1977	1978	1979
January	—	110	134	139	—	242	526	771
February	—	157	155	145	—	342	624	895
March	—	216	210	207	—	505	850	1,067
April	—	245	176	204	—	535	821	1,104
May	—	154	222	165	—	532	950	1,102
June	—	192	176	131	—	481	934	936
July	152	233	188	—	172	681	956	—
August	226	273	193	—	299	704	911	—
September	264	260	146	—	400	731	877	—
October	215	197	164	—	319	775	1,042	—
November	160	226	176	—	314	806	898	—
December	145	188	189	—	252	763	952	—
Total	1,162	2,451	2,129	2,500§	1,756	7,097	10,341	17,600§

*Medical care includes visits to physicians, nurse practitioner, nurse, and lab, x-ray and counselling services.
†First time enrollees at the health center.
‡Center opened July 1976.
§Total based on 6 months actual and 6 months projected.

while center expenses totaled $171,929. Approximately 16 percent of the center's gross charges were Medicaid-related.

The New Facility

The CMC was still in the Hemmingford storefront facility when 1977 ended. Selecting a site, securing a mortgage and designing the building had delayed construction until August 1977. The site selected was seven miles south of Hemmingford on a state highway and centrally located within the service area.

By the time construction began in August 1977, the original plans for a 3,200-square-foot building had evolved into a 7,000-square-foot facility with six exam rooms, offices, an x-ray room, a lab and a waiting room on the main floor and a dentist's office, five dental operatories, a reception area, classroom and storage and utility rooms on the basement level. The architect hired by the board, although experienced, was designing his first medical complex. Following a suggestion by one funding agency, an architect experienced in designing ambulatory care facilities was consulted by the board but could make only minor changes because construction was already under way.

The CMC soon discovered that building requirements accompanying Hill-Burton financing would place added burdens and delays on the project. As one illustration, Mr. Youngberg pointed to the $25,000 elevator installed in the two-story facility to satisfy Hill-Burton regulations. The cost of the elevator represented nearly one-quarter of the Hill-Burton funds made available to the CMC, and it usurped the space originally allocated for an exam room. Mr. Youngberg explained that the CMC had neglected to consider federal restrictions and their costs until the project was well under way.

Building delays had other ramifications. The passage of time meant higher construction costs. The final cost of the building (including equipment), originally planned at $353,596, was $741,488. Delays in occupying the new facility affected service expansions the CMC had planned, among them the addition of x-ray, complete laboratory, eye, mental health and physical therapy services. The CMC also had planned to initiate dental services in October 1977 to coincide with the move to the new facility.

In early 1978, the CMC decided to initiate the dental services without waiting for completion of the new center. The primary reason for this decision was that the center's second-year Rural Health Initiative grant had been awarded for dental services, and continued delays in expending those funds could result in their withdrawal. The board rented and remodeled a storefront facility adjoining the temporary Hemmingford medical center offices, hired Dr. Lowry Barnice and a dental hygienist and opened the temporary dental office in April 1978.

The new facility was completed in October 1978, one year behind schedule, and the temporary medical and dental offices in Hemmingford were vacated. Staff additions that coincided with the move to the new facility were a certified x-ray technician who was also to perform lab work, a part-time billing/insurance clerk, a part-time custodian, plus a receptionist/insurance clerk and two dental assistants for the dental practice *(Figure 3)*.

To keep pace with the staff expansions, Mr. Youngberg spent a good deal of time refining the CMC's personnel systems. New job descriptions, an employee grievance procedure and a wage and salary system were put into effect. A personnel committee of the board was responsible for approving these systems as well as any salary adjustments before final approval by the full board.

The National Health Service Corps Nurse Practitioner

In early 1978, Mr. Youngberg began encountering difficulties with Betty Ramsey, the National Health Service Corps nurse practitioner.

Figure 3 Community Medical Center Organizational Chart (October 1978)

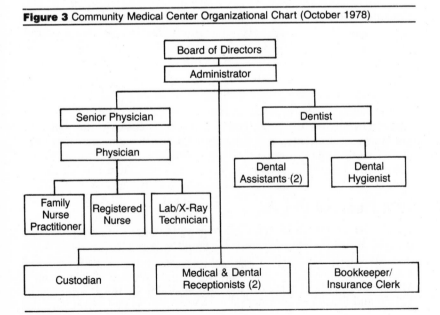

While both physicians were expected to utilize the nurse practitioner in the provision of patient care when appropriate, Dr. Kolb tended to use her less than Dr. Lee did. When absences or work loads warranted it, Mr. Youngberg occasionally assigned her duties typically performed by the center's nurse, such as preparing patients for the physicians and lab work. He discovered, however, that Mrs. Ramsey resisted these assignments and disliked performing nursing tasks at the center. Mr. Youngberg reported, "She soon began using the fact that she was an employee of the National Health Service Corps—and not directly a center employee—to circumvent me and undermine my authority. She also was unresponsive when I asked her to conduct educational programs at the center or in community locations, an activity the CMC had intended to inaugurate as part of the nurse practitioner's functions."

Mr. Youngberg decided to contact the CMC's designated project officer at the National Health Service Corps to find out whether he was placing realistic demands on the nurse practitioner. The project officer agreed with the alternative ways Mr. Youngberg suggested to utilize the nurse practitioner when necessitated by the center work load. Mr. Youngberg therefore continued his approach with the nurse practitioner and wrote a new job description for the role. However, Mrs. Ramsey found the job description unacceptable and complained to the regional office of the National Health Service Corps. In a reversal, the National Health Service Corps placed restrictions on what Mr. Youngberg could and could not expect the nurse practitioner to do: the nurse practitioner was to perform only direct patient care activities and could not be used in the lab or to prepare patients for the physicians.

The board became involved in the controversy and supported the administrator's decision that he could not work within the National Health Service Corps' restrictive guidelines. Mrs. Ramsey was discharged in September 1978. The board still supported the concept of nurse practitioner care and hoped to hire a new nurse practitioner directly rather than through the Corps when financial resources would permit (by July 1979).

1978 Financial Picture

At the end of 1978, the CMC was operating at approximately 51 percent self-sufficiency *(Figure 4)*. Patients were being charged the fees initially levied by the board in July 1976. The average cost per visit for all services was $26.10, while the average gross charge was $13.30. For medical care, the per-visit cost and charge averages were $21.75 and $11.43 and for dental care were $66.92 and $35 *(Figure 5)*.

Patient profiles for medical treatment showed that 76 percent of patients were billed for services either directly or through private insurers and 24 percent through Medicaid or Medicare.

The center collected 88 percent of its gross billings to self-pay patients in 1978. The board was responsible for setting the collection policy for self-pay patients, and an excerpt from the president's report at a board meeting illustrates the mechanisms used: "Letters to be sent to 14 patients who owe a total of $244.50 for collection. One to be notified they will no longer be treated here."

The center collected 58 percent of its gross billings to third parties during 1978. Under the state Medicaid program, the CMC was classified as a clinic, for which the fixed reimbursement rate was $9 per visit by a Medicaid-covered patient. Given the center's 1978 average cost per visit for medical care, a loss of nearly $13 was incurred on each visit by patients covered by Medicaid, who now constituted 22 percent of the CMC's patient volume. Compounding this reimbursement shortfall was a cash flow problem because Medicaid payments were not received until three to four months following billing.

Figure 4 Statement of Operating Income and Expenses*

	1/1/77– 12/31/77	1/1/78– 12/31/78	1/1/79– 12/31/79†
‡ **Income**			
Gross billings			
Medical			
Self-pay	$ 48,399	$ 62,494	$ 92,750
Medicare	—	1,843	3,500
Medicaid	12,490	26,391	38,500
Private insurance	17,174	27,476	40,250
Dental			
Self-pay	—	34,000	84,400
Total gross revenue	$ 78,063	$152,204	$259,400
Net revenue			
Medical			
Self-pay	$ 43,559	$ 55,425	$ 88,100
Medicare	—	} 32,422	} 65,800
Medicaid	} 18,914		
Private insurance			
Dental			
Self-pay	—	29,920	71,740
Total net revenue	$ 62,473	$117,767	$225,640

Expenses

Personnel

Physicians	$ 58,769	$ 80,000	$ 82,000
Nurse practitioner	5,500	11,000	15,000
Nurse	8,479	9,283	9,450
Aide	3,400	6,956	7,420
Administrator	15,596	17,000	17,850
Receptionist/bookkeeper	5,934	17,212	22,980§
Secretary	6,877	—	—
Janitor	723	1,749	3,000
Dentist	—	26,250	35,000
Dental assistants	—	4,160	16,640
Hygienist	—	9,000	13,000
Other	—	3,692	22,268
Fringe benefits	16,387	30,775	36,691
Total	$121,665	$217,077	$281,299

Non-personnel

Travel	$ 4,208	$ 3,241	$ 4,000
Office supplies	3,484	3,294	3,500
Medical supplies	7,446	8,218	8,500
Dental supplies	—	15,000	20,000
Rent, utilities, telephone, postage	8,201	21,735	48,000
Insurance	7,478	11,389	12,000
Radiology supplies	—	900	3,600
Other	19,447	17,742	10,000
Total	$ 50,264	$ 81,519	$109,600
Total expenses	$171,929	$298,596	$390,899

*Numbers have been rounded.
†Projected income and expenses.
‡Expenses not covered by patient revenue were subsidized by grants.
§Four individuals: two full-time, two part-time.

Similarly, Medicare reimbursement, although applicable to only about two percent of the 1978 gross billings, was based on restrictive profiles and generally did not cover the full amount of charges.

Focus on Fiscal Improvement

Although administrator Youngberg attributed the CMC's current financial picture primarily to recent facility and service expansion costs, he knew he had to find a way to improve the center's revenue-to-cost ratio and begin achieving a greater degree of financial solvency. He also suspected that the center's financial condition and recent community complaints about long waits for appointments might be related. These complaints had been made directly to board

Figure 5 Expense and Income Summary by Cost Center–1/1/78-12/31/78

	A	B	C	D	E	F*
Provider Services Functional Cost Center	Patient Visits	Salaries	Consultants & Contracts	Supplies	Total Direct Expense (B+C+D)	Fringe Benefits (indirect expense)
Physicians	8,360	79,999.92		8,218.38	88,218.30	17,849.49
Nurse Practitioner	1,586	11,000.00			11,000.00	2,461.99
Laboratory	32	1,846.00	1,250.20		3,096.20	307.75
X-Ray	3	1,846.00	905.50	900.00	3,651.50	307.75
Dental	1,100	39,410.00		15,000.00	54,410.00	8,924.76
Counseling	360	4,641.37			4,641.37	923.25
Total Provider Services	11,441	138,743.29	2,155.70	24,118.38	165,017.37	30,774.99

*Allocation to cost center based on cost center's percentage of total salary expense applied to total fringe benefit expense.

Figure 5 Expense and Income Summary by Cost Center (Cont'd)

	G†	H	I	J	K
Provider Services Functional Cost Center	Maintenance & Support Services (indirect expense)	Total Expense (E+F+G)	Gross Charges	Average Cost per Visit	Percent Cost Covered by Charges
Physicians	75,045.83	181,113.62	99,078.20	21.66	54.7%
Nurse Practitioner	14,392.35	27,854.34	17,446.00	17.56	62.6%
Laboratory	514.01	3,917.96	165.00	122.44	4.0%
X-Ray	514.01	4,473.26	75.00	1,491.08	2.0%
Dental	10,280.25	73,615.01	34,000.00	66.92	46.2%
Counseling	2,056.05	7,620.67	1,440.00	21.17	18.9%
Total Provider Services	102,802.50	298,594.86	152,204.20	26.10	50.9%

†Allocation to cost center based on cost center's percentage of total patient visits applied to total maintenance and support services expense. Maintenance and Support Services consists of $72,603.10 support services expense and $30,199.40 building and maintenance expense. Total indirect expense (F + G) equals $133,577.49.

members, and the board in turn had referred them to Mr. Youngberg. Although the complaints seemed to end after the administrator contacted the individuals and explained that the medical center had been particularly busy because of the flu season, Mr. Youngberg wondered if they signalled a more serious problem.

Mr. Youngberg discussed the complaints with the two physicians, who proposed adding a third physician. Mr. Youngberg knew that the CMC could not afford a third physician since the center was only generating enough revenue to cover 51 percent of its costs.

Looking for possible causes for the occasional overcrowding of the center and possible solutions to the center's revenue problems, Mr. Youngberg focused on three factors: the fees charged for services rendered, physician productivity and physician charge patterns. Because of the sensitive nature of these issues and his own limited experience, Mr. Youngberg obtained a consultant, Frank Montana, to aid his investigation.

Fees

The CMC's administrator had been convinced for some time that the center's fee schedule was low in view of the cost of providing the services, the prices charged by other physicians in the area and reimbursement shortfalls. The board, however, was reluctant to increase fees for fear of the possible effect on utilization of the center.

In April 1979, with the help of Mr. Montana, Mr. Youngberg succeeded in convincing the board to raise fees, and the first increase since the center opened was instituted. The CMC began charging $6 for a brief visit, $12 for a basic visit and $18 for an extended visit with a physician. Ancillary fees were raised an average of 25 percent. Although the center's $12 charge for a basic visit was competitive at the time, area physicians were raising their fees at a faster rate, so the CMC's charges soon fell below the average for the area. Shortly after the CMC raised its fees, the state raised the Medicaid reimbursement for clinic visits to $15, or $3 more than the center's charge for a basic visit.

Physician Productivity and Charge Patterns

Mr. Youngberg and Mr. Montana also examined the center's utilization in relationship to revenues generated. The data showed that the center's average annual encounters (4,180 per physician) approached the norm set by the Rural Health Initiative program (4,200 per year).

The data also showed that Dr. Kolb and Dr. Lee saw nearly the same number of patients. However, Dr. Kolb maintained this productivity level only by working extra hours on his own. Described by Mr. Youngberg as a very thorough physician, Dr. Kolb typically scheduled no more than three patients per hour and spent about one-quarter of his time charting. The young physician liked to establish personal rapport with his patients and spend more time with them than the typical visit schedule allowed. When Mr. Youngberg questioned him about his practice style, Dr. Kolb responded that quality of care would suffer if he scheduled more patients per hour than was his custom. Since Dr. Kolb was willing to work extra hours and thereby achieve a productivity level comparable to that of Dr. Lee, Mr. Youngberg felt that he could not take issue on that basis.

In monitoring the gross charges corresponding to the patient visits, however, Mr. Youngberg identified an obvious difference between the two physicians *(Figure 6)*. Despite a comparable number of patient visits, Dr. Kolb was generating less revenue because of his reluctance to adhere to the established fee schedule.

Mr. Youngberg also believed that, while some of the center's patient overload could be attributed to the loss of the nurse practitioner, who typically saw 20 to 25 patients a day, physician productivity was partly to blame as well.

As Mr. Youngberg began to work with Mr. Montana to formulate a plan for addressing these physician issues, however, a series of crises arose that diverted his attention.

Figure 6 Patient Visits and Gross Charges by Physician–1/79-6/79

	Patient Visits		Gross Charges	
	Dr. Kolb	Dr. Lee	Dr. Kolb	Dr. Lee
January	501	210*	$ 5,468	$ 2,952
February	356	391	4,186	5,527
March	421	548	4,565	7,654
April	473	473	5,407	7,910
May	407	493	5,106	7,529
June	343	423	4,063	6,657
Total	2,501	2,538	$28,795	$38,229

*Dr. Lee on vacation for two weeks.

Adverse Publicity

In the late spring of 1979, the CMC again encountered criticism from patients. This time it began with letters to the local newspaper in which several patients complained that appointments were needed to receive care, that emergency cases were sometimes referred to a hospital, that the center was not open 24 hours a day and that the fees were too high. These charges stimulated newspaper articles, and several members of the town council went on record as opposing the center's practices.

To Mr. Youngberg and the board, these charges indicated a misunderstanding of the center's purposes. The CMC countered them, explaining in newspaper articles that misinterpretation and misunderstanding of the center's purpose, and not deficiency in services or practices, were causing the patient dissatisfaction. Mr. Youngberg acknowledged that a statement in the center's brochure, listing "24-hour full coverage" as a CMC goal, had been interpreted by patients to mean the center was open around the clock. Mr. Youngberg also felt that the community apparently viewed the center as a "clinic," providing free or reduced-cost care, a view he believed was reinforced by the center's request for charitable support from the community and by its charter as a community corporation.

Disruption in Dental Services

During this period of patient and public criticism, Dr. Barnice, the center dentist who had completed one year of a three-year contract, requested a new contract with a raise of 8½ percent for each of the two remaining years. His annual salary was $35,000 under a contract that included no increases. The board refused the dentist's demands but offered him an alternate contract with an 8½ percent increase for both years. Dr. Barnice found the offer unacceptable and went on strike for five days. When the board refused to change its position, Dr. Barnice quit, rented a nearby facility and opened a private practice. This represented another violation of the contract, which contained a provision prohibiting the dentist from practicing independently in the center's service area for one year after leaving the CMC. The board decided to initiate legal action against Dr. Barnice.

In the interim, however, Mr. Youngberg was faced with patients scheduled for dental services. He knew he had to find a resolution quickly or incur more dissatisfaction from patients and possible irreparable damage to the center's image. By this time, the second half of 1979 was approaching and Mr. Youngberg was concerned about the

CMC's fiscal position, particularly since major operational grants from the Hospital Research and Educational Trust and the Rural Health Initiative program had recently expired. However, several obstacles seemed to be preventing the CMC from accomplishing financial self-sufficiency, among them a full patient schedule that underutilized the facility and its equipment, the sudden departure of the center's only dentist, problems with physician productivity and community criticism of center practices.

Exhibit Employment Contract

Employee contract between Community Medical Center of Northwest Delaware County, Inc. and

_____, M.D.

Whereas, the Community Medical Center of Northwest Delaware County, Inc., hereinafter referred to as the Center, is a non-profit public corporation founded in 1973 to provide primary health services to the residents of: Northwest Delaware County, to include the Revoso, Hemmingford, and Fort Dodge School Districts. At a facility located at 430 South Main Street, Hemmingford, soon to be located on Route 25 between Hemmingford and Delaware, Delaware County, Ohio.

And Whereas, _____ M.D., hereinafter referred to as the Physician, is a physician licensed to practice medicine in Ohio.

Therefore be it Resolved:

Term of this Agreement

The period covered by this contract shall be from July 8, 1977 to July 7, 1980. This contract shall automatically be renewed for an additonal three year period ending July 7, 1983 unless written notice to the contrary is transmitted from one party to the other no less than ninety (90) days prior to the termination of the first period.

Remuneration of Physician

The Center shall remunerate the Physician at the rate of $19.23 per hour of service. The Center hereby guarantees the Physician no less than 2,080 hours of service per year for a total gross earnings of $39,998 per year. The Physician's contributions to Social Security, Withholding Taxes, and any other deductions required by law or authorized by the Physician shall be withheld by the Center.

Working Hours

The Center shall be open to the public for a minimum of 40 hours and a maximum of 80 hours per week. Patients will be seen 3-6 evenings a week from 6:00 p.m. to 9:00 p.m. and on Saturdays from 9:00 a.m. to 5:00 p.m. The Physician will provide a minimum of 40 hours and a maximum of 50 hours of patient care per week including a minimum of 8 and a maximum of 14 hours per two weeks of service during evening and Saturday office hours.

Fringe Benefits   The Center shall provide the Physician with the following:

a)   21 days paid vacation per year.

b)   5 days of continuing education with pay and reimbursement per year. (up to $500/yr.)

c)   12 days sick leave with pay per year. (Those days not used on or before the annual anniversary date of this contract are forfeited.)

d)   9½ paid holidays as follows:

New Year's Day   Veterans Day
Washington's Birthday   Independence Day
Memorial Day   Thanksgiving & the day after
Labor Day   Christmas & ½ day prior

e)   Blue Cross and Blue Shield Family Coverage

1.   Major Medical Insurance
2.   Disability Insurance

f) $50,000.00 of Term Life Insurance

g)   Personal Days: three authorized absences with pay for personal reasons will be allowed each year. Prior approval is needed and subject to the following:

a)   usable for observance of religious holidays such as Good Friday, holy days of obligation, Rosh Hashanah, Yom Kippur, etc...

b)   usable any day which is normally considered a working day.

Personal days may not be considered as part of a scheduled vacation or in conjunction with any of the established holidays. They should be taken separately except when consecutive religious holidays require it. Personal days are not accumulative from year to year.

Liability Insurance   The Center shall pay for 100% of the Physician's professional liability insurance totaling not less than $100,000 with a $300,000 "umbrella" or a "catastrophic" clause. The physician shall pay for any insurance that is not necessary for his normal duties at the Center.

Relocation Expenses   The Center will reimburse the Physician for all expenses incurred in relocating his household to the service area of the Center for an amount not to exceed $200.

Place of Residence   The Physician, it is hoped, will live within the service area of the Center. The Center hereby agrees to assist, to the fullest extent possible, in locating suitable housing and arranging the necessary financing.

Exclusiveness of Services   The Physician hereby agrees that he will not offer his professional services elsewhere in the trade area covered by the Center which would duplicate those he is providing at the Center during the term of this agreement. This does not include admitting Center patients to the hospital or hospital emergency room work, providing it does not interfere with the Medical Center's schedule. The Physician further agrees not to offer professional services which would duplicate those he provides at the Center within a period of one (1) year from the expiration of this agreement, within the Center's service area.

Equipment & Supplies

All necessary equipment and supplies, both expendable and nonexpendable drugs, furniture, and fixtures which are required for the efficient operation of a primary health care center shall be provided by the Center. Included in this would be laboratory coats or other uniforms selected by the physician to be worn while performing his duties. The administration of the Center shall solicit recommendations from the Physician prior to purchasing equipment and new supply items.

Maintenance & Repair

The Center shall maintain and repair all equipment and shall provide utilities and services such as heat, water, electricity, telephone services, laundry, janitorial service, painting, and decorating.

Nurses & Auxiliary Personnel

The Center shall provide the services of such nurses and auxiliary personnel as are essential for efficient and competent clinic operations.

Medical Records

The Physician shall maintain adequate medical records for all of his patients utilizing forms provided by the Center. These records shall remain the property of the Center upon termination of this contract.

Billing of Patients

No patient shall receive services at a rate other than that set by the Board of Directors. Patients shall be billed by the Center and all receipts shall be the property of the Center. (This excludes billing of patients in the hospital and other billings not associated with the Center).

Administration

The Board of Directors of the Center retain legal, fiscal, and administrative responsibility for the operation of the Center. The administrator of the Center shall act as the sole agent of the Board of Directors and shall be responsible for implementing its directives. The physician shall defer to the judgment of the administrator in all non-clinical matters (e.g. the setting of fees, purchase of equipment, hiring of personnel). The Center, through the administrator, shall provide ample opportunity (through staff meetings, etc.) for the physician to express his opinion on major administrative proposals prior to their implementation. The Physician agrees to respect the organizational structure.

Clinical Integrity

The Center shall defer to the judgment of the Physician on all clinical matters (e.g. the diagnosis and treatment of disease). While the physician shall make every effort to practice medicine in harmony with the administrative policy and procedures of the Center, his responsibility to the patient shall predominate in all instances.

Clinical Procedures

The Physician shall conform to all such uniform Clinical protocols and procedures which may be established by his medical peers.

Clinical Evaluation

The Center shall establish a systematic and periodic program of clinical evaluation utilizing the services of physicians not practicing at the Center. The Physician shall cooperate fully in all such matters. The Center agrees that these evaluations shall be confidential and constructive in intent and purpose and fully integrated with the Center's continuing education program.

Cooperation in Surveys

The Physician recognizes that the Center has certain obligations to provide information to other public agencies including: the Ohio Department of Health, the Hill-Burton Program, and the National Health Service Corps. The Center will attempt to minimize inconvenience to the Physician in complying with all such requests. The Physician agrees to supply the information and opinions solicited.

Independent Research & Publication

The Physician is free to contribute clinical articles, with or without remuneration, to medical and research periodicals, text books, etc., so long as this work does not interfere with routine clinical responsibilities. The Physician agrees, however, not to use other than accepted clinical procedures in the course of his research without the explicit consent of the medical director. The convenience, comfort, and privacy of the patients shall be respected at all times. All articles concerning the design, planning and administration of health centers shall be submitted to the administrator for review and comment prior to publication.

Operating Procedure

The Physician agrees to adhere to all aspects of the Center's written operating procedures where these are not in conflict with the terms of this contract or generally accepted clinical practice.

Termination of Contract

This contract shall be automatically voided if at anytime during the period covered by this contract:

a) The Physician forfeits his license to practice medicine within Ohio.

b) The Center should be required for reasons beyond its control to terminate operation.

c) This contract may be voluntarily terminated if agreed to by both parties.

Settlement of Disputes

In the event that any dispute shall arise between the Center and the Physician concerning the provisions and terms of this Contract, both parties hereby agree that the matter shall be presented to the Executive-Personnel Committees or the Board of Directors of the Center before any other action is taken. Presentation of the dispute to the Committees or Board for decision is hereby declared a condition precedent to any legal action by either party of this agreement.

9
Montgomery County Hospital

Montgomery County Hospital

Introduction

Two rural primary care health centers—one in Biscoe and the other in Warner-Robbins—were scheduled to open in July 1977. The centers, satellites of Montgomery County Hospital in Seagrove, a small Southern city *(Figure 1)*, were being funded through federal and private grants to the hospital totaling $252,000.* Although the hospital planned to operate the centers, advisory boards in each community were to work with the hospital in developing the centers. One year later, in July 1978, opening of the Warner-Robbins center was nowhere in sight. The Biscoe center was closer to being a reality but still had not opened for lack of physician resources. The Biscoe center finally opened in October 1978, but its first seven months were characterized by low utilization and a poor financial condition.

Calvin Chapelwaite, president of Montgomery County Hospital since its opening in 1971, talked about how the idea of the centers originated:

> There's no debating the fact that the hospital's enabling legislation mandated that the hospital do its part to improve access to primary care in Montgomery County. However, I didn't believe it was the hospital's responsibility to construct and operate rural primary care facilities. We started getting pressure to do that, though. In 1974, county officials threatened to deny the hospital the tax funds allocated for the care of the indigent, which was a fairly substantial amount, if we didn't do something to help the medically underserved communities. The communities themselves were putting similar pressure on the hospital's board of trustees. The board couldn't ignore those people because they controlled the purse strings when the hospital needed tax allocations or bond financing.

---

*A two-year, $150,000 grant from the Hospital Research and Educational Trust and a one-year, $102,000 federal grant from the Rural Health Initiative program.

Figure 1 Montgomery County

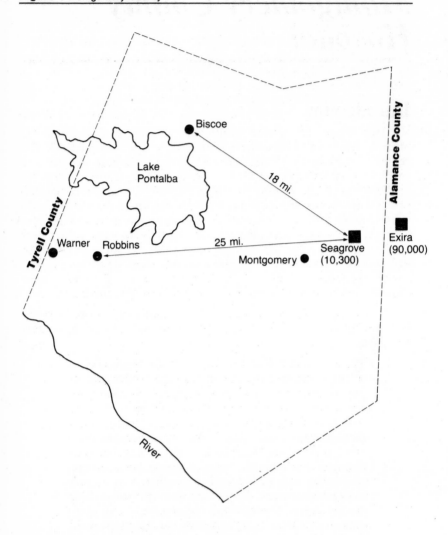

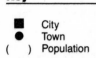

In 1975, the county had created a task force to make some recommendations based on county health needs. Montgomery County Hospital president Chapelwaite appointed his administrative assistant, Janice Decina, to be the hospital's liaison with the task force. Among its findings, the task force had identified Biscoe, with a service area population of 11,000, and Warner-Robbins, with a service area population of 13,000, as prime locations for hospital satellite clinics. According to Miss Decina, two other factors entered into the hospital's decision to establish satellite centers: the rural communities were unable to attract private practice physicians, and federal and private funds were available for primary care center initiatives. Mr. Chapelwaite also felt that it was important for Montgomery County Hospital to establish itself as a forward-looking institution in order to keep pace with Alamance Memorial Hospital, a county facility in nearby Exira (in Alamance County).

Despite the hospital's intentions and the existence of financial resources, progress on the centers was negligible. In explaining this situation, Mr. Chapelwaite cited a number of reasons:

> For every family practitioner completing training in the state, I'd estimate there were 10 job opportunities in the state, most in population centers with hospitals and cultural activity. In trying to set up the centers, Montgomery County Hospital was competing for recruits against physician groups who were offering established practices and proximity to a hospital. In comparison, we were offering an unproven practice located up to 25 miles from the hospital.

> There were other complications as well. We had to devote a lot of time and energy to working with the community groups to form advisory boards. We also had to contend with various demands the communities levied—such as no foreign medical graduates. Another problem I was working on was the negative reaction of the Montgomery County Hospital medical staff to the whole idea of the hospital setting up the primary care centers. We needed the medical staff's support to entice physicians to the centers and to give them admitting privileges at the hospital.

> We did have these difficulties to deal with, but so would anyone in the same situation. They may have slowed us down but were by no means insurmountable.

Stephen Walsh, who chaired the Warner-Robbins community coalition that was working with the hospital in opening that community's center, had a different explanation for the inability to attract physicians to rural communities. He believed that the medical education system made physicians overly dependent on hospital facilities. Mr. Walsh observed that the hospital was encountering the same problem the community had faced for years: potential physician recruits rejecting job offers because their practice would be "too far from the hospital." Mr. Walsh's view of the medical education system was that it trained doctors to rely on highly advanced technology and hospital resources rather than developing self-reliance.

Montgomery County Hospital

Montgomery County, a predominantly rural area except for Seagrove at its extreme eastern end, was the state's fastest growing county during the 1970s. In 1962, the citizens of Montgomery County voted to construct a county hospital to serve all residents, including the 32 percent who were indigent. With the defeat of a bond issue in 1964, however, the hospital did not begin taking shape until a private citizen donated 23 acres of land near Seagrove for the facility. The General Assembly originally had contemplated locating the hospital near the town of Montgomery.

Following a series of General Assembly actions, including mandates that the county hospital assist in the provision of primary care throughout the county and that it utilize community advisory boards, Montgomery County Hospital opened in 1971. By 1972, occupancy was at 90 percent and the care provided was referral/specialist-oriented.* Services such as x-ray and laboratory were the only ones provided on an outpatient basis. In 1977, following a $10-million expansion financed by a county bond issue, the hospital had 248 beds and a relatively young (average age of 40) medical staff.

Montgomery County Hospital Medical Staff

The county hospital's medical staff consisted of 170 fee-for-service physicians, plus five emergency room physicians who were on contract full-time. The emergency room physicians were paid a salary, which was supplemented by a percentage of the hospital's charge to any

---

*Specialists with active status included: three anesthesiologists, two dermatologists, two ear, nose and throat specialists, three general practitioners, four internists, four obstetrician/gynecologists, two ophthalmologists, nine orthopedic surgeons, two pathologists, three pediatricians, three radiologists, fifteen surgeons, one plastic surgeon, seven urologists and five emergency room physicians.

patients they treated in the emergency room above a specified number. Samuel O'Connor, M.D., was chief of staff and Ralph Loeffler, M.D., was chief of the emergency staff.

The medical staff was organized according to three classifications that governed staff privileges: active, courtesy and consulting. The 65 physicians with active privileges had no restrictions on the number of patients they could admit to the hospital, but were required to provide on-call emergency room coverage on a rotating basis. Members with courtesy privileges could admit one patient per month and were not required to provide emergency room coverage. Physicians with consulting privileges could admit one patient per year. The 110 courtesy and consulting staff had primary affiliations with other hospitals and typically had practices distant from Seagrove.

Biscoe and Warner-Robbins

Biscoe is a small but fast-growing resort community 18 miles (by interstate highway) west of Seagrove on the northern edge of Lake Pontalba that attracts many summer visitors and residents. Many of Biscoe's 400 permanent residents commute the 20 miles to Exira, the state capital, for employment. There were no physicians practicing in Biscoe in 1976.

Warner and Robbins are two adjoining communities separated by 300 barren yards and situated across the lake from Biscoe. Unlike Biscoe, the Warner-Robbins area, with a population of 5,000, was described as stagnant. There was a long history of competition between the two towns of Warner and Robbins, stemming from a debate over whether to merge the two towns or maintain them as separate entities. The only full-time physician in the area was Alex Perlman, M.D., who had set up practice there in 1963. Two other physicians were elderly and practiced only part-time.

Plans for the Primary Care Centers

When Montgomery County Hospital decided to establish the two primary care centers, Mr. Chapelwaite assigned the project to Stacy Tandrell, a recent state university graduate holding an M.B.A. with a health emphasis, who had been hired by Mr. Chapelwaite in 1976 as assistant for special projects. Janice Decina, Mr. Chapelwaite's administrative assistant, worked closely with Mr. Tandrell in laying the groundwork for the hospital's satellite center project and applying for the grants to finance it.

The hospital's proposal to the grant agencies for developing the two primary care centers outlined the responsibilities of all parties concerned—the communities, the hospital and the center physicians. Community involvement in the form of advisory boards was already mandated in the hospital's enabling legislation. As outlined by the hospital, each community was to provide an appropriate facility to house its center, nominate consumer advisory board members for approval by the hospital board of trustees, advise the hospital in matters pertaining to center administration and help determine who the management should be after the grants expired. The hospital, as manager, was responsible for all medical and financial aspects of the project, including employing and compensating staff, billing, purchasing and quality control. Any revenues exceeding expenses were to be applied solely to the hospital's primary care delivery system in the county. Eligible family practitioners for the centers must have completed residency training in family medicine, be certified to practice in the state and have active status on the Montgomery County Hospital medical staff. The decision to give the center physicians active medical staff status was based on research studies showing that a physician's hospital practice is an important part of a primary care center's income. With active status, the center physicians would be required to share rotating on-call coverage in the hospital's emergency room. The physicians would be retained on contract with the hospital at a set annual salary of $48,000 and would be encouraged, but not required, to reside in the respective communities.

Each satellite would be staffed by two family practice physicians, a family nurse practitioner, a registered nurse, a nursing assistant, a laboratory technician and a receptionist/bookkeeper. The centers would be open during daytime hours, and the hospital expected the physicians at each center to be responsible for after-hours coverage of their patients.

From Plans to Action

It was Stacy Tandrell's responsibility to execute the plans for setting up primary care centers in Biscoe and Warner-Robbins.

Mr. Tandrell's efforts to recruit physicians began in March 1977 and encompassed contacts with the state medical association's Rural Health Delivery Project, the U.S. Public Health Service's National Health Manpower Shortage Clearinghouse, the Area Health Education Center Physician Recruitment Program in Asheville, nine private placement agencies and all seven state family practice training programs, where program directors reported that most graduating residents were already committed to practices. In all, he contacted more than 50 physicians in an attempt to recruit for the satellites.

Two residents expressed an interest. Peter Kistner, M.D., a third-year resident in Exira, was interested in the Biscoe center. Initial contacts between Dr. Kistner, the hospital and representatives from Biscoe resulted in the drafting of a contract between the hospital and Dr. Kistner. The other potential candidate was Paul Gregerson, M.D., a second-year resident in Exira. He also expressed an interest in the Biscoe center and agreed to negotiate a contract. He would be able to begin practice upon completion of his residency in July 1978.

Also expressing an interest was Dr. Perlman, the physician practicing in Warner-Robbins. Dr. Perlman was not on the Montgomery County Hospital medical staff but had taken an active role in the Warner-Robbins community group working with the hospital on the center project. He was considering accepting one of the physician positions at the Warner-Robbins center and also offered his offices as a temporary site for the center. He stipulated, however, that he would not accept the post if he were the only physician at the center.

In addition to recruiting physicians, Mr. Tandrell also was working with the communities, where progress was limited and several months behind schedule. A Biscoe advisory board had been organized, had raised $30,000 to lease a building and had plans ready for renovating it. Warner-Robbins had not yet formed an advisory board, but a nonprofit community corporation was serving in its place temporarily. The group had rented but not yet renovated a former funeral home for the center. (Dr. Perlman's office was too small.)

Mr. Tandrell believed that the major reason for the delay in organizing the centers was his inability to recruit physicians. Of the three possibilities identified so far, one was already practicing in the community, one would not be available until mid-1978 and the third seemed to be vacillating in his decision to sign a contract.

Mr. Tandrell explained what he thought was behind the questionable physician recruitment results: "A large part of it was the attitude of the Montgomery County Hospital medical staff. They seemed to be opposed to the hospital's plans to set up the satellite centers, but I wasn't privy to what was going on. At some point, Mr. Chapelwaite had decided to take certain matters into his own hands, particularly dealing with the medical staff, which left me at a disadvantage in being able to fit all the pieces together."

Medical Staff Concerns

Dr. O'Connor's appointment as chief of staff had not yet taken effect when the hospital submitted its grant application in 1976. Although his predecessor had signed the application, Dr. O'Connor, as chief-designate, had been consulted. Mr. Chapelwaite therefore was surprised when he began hearing strong opposition from the medical staff shortly after the physician recruitment efforts for the centers began. Both Dr. O'Connor and Dr. Loeffler approached the hospital's president with an assortment of protests. Dr. Loeffler, the hospital's emergency room chief, was the most upset. In a private meeting with Mr. Chapelwaite, Dr. Loeffler said :

> Some of my staff have serious reservations about the kind of operation that is being planned for Biscoe and Warner. We have all we can handle in the emergency room right now and I'm really worried that the physicians out there are going to tax our capacity. After all, the offices out there are only going to be open from nine to five. After five, those patients are going to want to be seen at the emergency room if they have a problem. The emergency room is going to be turned into an after-hours 'convenience' for the center physicians.

In response, Mr. Chappelwaite reminded Dr. Loeffler that a considerable portion of the Biscoe residents already used the emergency room for general illnesses and that starting the centers, at least in Biscoe, should lighten the emergency room's nonemergency load. Dr. Loeffler rebutted with: "It's correct that we see some patients from those areas right now for less than a true emergency, but at least we're able to work them in around the true emergencies, especially since we know who we've asked to come back and for what reason. We'll have no way to predict what the volume is likely to be. My staff physicians are not too pleased about this whole deal." Mr. Chapelwaite replied:

> I can certainly understand your concerns, Dr. Loeffler. This project does have some problems, but I think we are working them out one by one and I'm glad you've taken this opportunity to talk with me. Our tentative contract for the health center physicians clearly requires the physicians to be responsible for their own patients after hours. As a matter of fact, that's why we're interested in having two physicians out there—so they will be able to share after-hour calls. I would be happy to have you review the contract, which we modeled after your own by the way, and make suggestions to me about changes you think are necessary. Perhaps you would like me to review your own contract and see if there's a way we can assure you that this initiative won't hurt your

contract arrangements. Let's keep in touch and see if we can't resolve these concerns.

A few days later, Dr. O'Connor also met with Mr. Chapelwaite concerning the health center physicians. Dr. O'Connor said:

You know, Calvin, the last medical staff meeting we had got pretty hot about the hospital's plans. I have to tell you that I'm against what you're doing out there. We're against the federal and state government doing it and now suddenly our own hospital is doing it. A lot of the staff see the hospital as setting a bad precedent by setting up private medical practices. It just sounds a whole lot like the beginnings of socialized medicine. Now I'm not saying *you* would do this, but the next thing you know, somebody will be telling the rest of us physicians who we can and can't admit to the hospital.

Dr. O'Connor went on to say:

The staff has another serious concern. The private practice physicians north of Biscoe reportedly aren't happy with the idea of a Biscoe health center. There are rumors that they might start referring their patients to Alamance Memorial's medical staff instead of here. Also, most of the physicians you're interviewing for those centers were trained at Alamance Memorial, and I'll bet they'll refer their patients there rather than to us. Now nobody's going to like that.

I'll tell you another thing, Calvin. Physicians on salary are trouble. I know from my own experience at an Office of Economic Opportunity clinic that they just don't care as much. Why should they? They're getting a set salary whether they see nine or 30 patients. Just look at the demands one of the candidates for the center made: a starting salary of $75,000, eight-hour days and no on-call duty. All of us here today really had to struggle to start out in practice, but you're handing everything to these boys on a silver platter.

Mr. Chapelwaite replied:

I can certainly appreciate the points you've made, Dr. O'Connor, but there are some things I can probably clear up for you. First, the hospital is only going to be sponsoring these centers for two years.

After this grant money runs out, I fully intend that either the physicians or the communities themselves will take over their operation. Even though the hospital is involved, I have made a firm commitment not to use hospital funds for these centers. They are going to have to make it on their own. I was getting a lot of pressure from both the communities and the legislature to do something in these areas. I was under the threat of fund cuts. You can see what that would do to this hospital and to your own staff practices. My hands are tied. This was the option I thought would involve the hospital for the shortest length of time and satisfy both the communities and the legislature.

Second, the studies Janice Decina did before this plan even got off the ground showed that referrals to all of you should actually increase. One of the things we've considered putting in the physician contracts is a provision requiring them to use Montgomery County Hospital as their chief place of referral. Even though we initially said that these physicians should have active privileges here, I'd settle for your simply giving them courtesy privileges. That way, they would have to refer their patients and they'd be no different from any of the other physicians from that area. They wouldn't be getting any special treatment compared with any other outlying physician.

I can understand your feelings, Dr. O'Connor, but I really hope you can see your way clear to working with us on this project. If you think it would help, I'd be glad to meet with the medical staff or set up a meeting between you and the physicians we are considering.

Based on these conversations, Mr. Chapelwaite believed that the medical staff's opposition to the project resulted largely from misunderstandings and feelings of resentment and would have to be handled with caution and skill. Seeing it as a potentially volatile issue, the chief executive officer decided to handle it personally while letting Mr. Tandrell attend to the other details of organizing the centers.

Drs. O'Connor and Loeffler continued to pressure the president to abandon the project, at least in the form conceptualized. Dr. O'Connor set up a meeting of the medical staff leadership, Mr. Chapelwaite and the hospital board chairman at a nearby retreat to argue for abandoning the project. When that failed, the medical staff attempted to influence the hospital's plans in other ways. They placed restrictions on the types of physicians they would allow on staff, refusing to accept an osteopath for example. Rumors circulated that medical staff members were contacting potential recruits to persuade them not to appear for interviews.

In addition, Mr. Chapelwaite's proposal to Dr. O'Connor that the center physicians be accorded courtesy privileges by the medical staff was thwarted when the medical staff found a bylaws provision under which they could deny courtesy status to physicians without active status elsewhere. The likelihood that the center physicians could maintain active status at another hospital was remote, given the locations and arrangements associated with the centers. Mr. Chapelwaite arranged to have an independent physician consultant meet with the medical staff to address their concerns. The medical staff boycotted two such scheduled meetings.

Mr. Chapelwaite finally managed to arrange a meeting among himself, Dr. Loeffler and Dr. Gregerson, one of the Biscoe physician recruits, hoping that it would alleviate some of the concerns of the emergency room chief. Mr. Chapelwaite reported that "things seemed to quiet down" after that meeting. Dr. Gregerson, however, was not convinced that the emergency room staff's opposition had subsided. He believed that the main reason for Dr. Loeffler's opposition was the centers' potential effect on the incentive income of the emergency room staff. He felt that no amount of convincing or compromising by the hospital president would overcome that basic concern.

Center Progress

While Mr. Chapelwaite was addressing the concerns of the medical staff, Mr. Tandrell was attending to the other activities associated with development of the centers. As of July 1977, he also had a new position—administrative director of ambulatory services. In addition to working on the centers, he now carried administrative responsibilities for the emergency room and outpatient services at Montgomery County Hospital.

Mr. Tandrell's progress in the satellite center project was being hampered by both ongoing and newly emerging problems revolving around physician recruitment, the communities and confusion about his own administrative role in the project.

First, physician recruitment efforts were still largely unsuccessful. One of the physicians Mr. Tandrell was trying to recruit for the project did not want active privileges at Montgomery County Hospital because that required sharing on-call coverage at the emergency room, which was 45 minutes away from the center site. The physician wanted courtesy status, which would give him affiliation and admitting privileges without emergency room coverage duties. Mr. Chapelwaite had already proposed this arrangement in his negotiations with the medical staff, although Mr. Tandrell was unaware of it.

Dr. Perlman, the Warner-Robbins physician who was negotiating a contract with the hospital, had several concerns that made him reluctant to sign. He believed the primary care centers should provide comprehensive care but thought the hospital expected them to render episodic care, similar to the Montgomery County Hospital emergency room philosophy. Although he was not sure of what the future would hold for the centers, Dr. Perlman doubted that they could survive independently given the number of indigent in the service area. He also refused to sign a contract until a second physician was recruited for the center. So far, no candidate had signed a contract.

Second, the communities, although supportive and enthusiastic about the prospect of the centers, were presenting Mr. Tandrell with another set of problems. The Warner-Robbins group was in a continual state of fluctuation and could not seem to organize into a functional and cohesive advisory board. Both communities were making slow progress in securing facilities and were more of a hindrance than a help in the physician recruitment process, demanding that the center physicians reside in the community and refusing to accept a foreign medical graduate.

Third, Mr. Tandrell was confronted with growing confusion about the project and about several recent moves by Mr. Chapelwaite. This confusion stemmed from Mr. Tandrell's inability to gain access to and information from the president, which he felt was necessary to his job. As Mr. Tandrell illustrated:

> In the beginning, I had good access to Mr. Chapelwaite through Janice, so I knew what his goals were and could go there for help in addressing administrative questions. However, when Janice resigned her post [about six months after the grant started], I lost that access. Mr. Chapelwaite left all the administrative details up to me because that wasn't his strength or his area of interest, yet he continued to step in with alternate plans and decisions. My problem was I didn't know what his motives were or how I was supposed to go about implementing these new directions.

Changes in Direction

In December 1977, Mr. Chapelwaite made two decisions that he hoped would alter the stagnant course of the satellite project. First, he decided that the hospital should retrench into a supportive role with the community groups assuming greater responsibility, principally for physician recruitment. He believed this approach would placate the medical staff while still meeting the needs of the hospital and the communities. It also would head the project in the direction demanded by the Rural Health Initiative program, which was increasing the pressure for community board rather than hospital sponsorship of the centers. Mr. Chapelwaite also believed that, for the recruitment efforts to succeed, the communities would need to do more to promote themselves to potential candidates, an approach he said the hospital had been remiss in not encouraging. Second, he increased Mr. Tandrell's time allocation to the project so that he could assist the communities in the recruitment process and in the administrative details of organizing into fully functional boards.

The communities did not react favorably to the idea of being given more responsibility for the project, particularly for the physician recruitment process. They expected the hospital to recruit the physicians for the centers because they interpreted that to fall under the hospital's mandate to improve the delivery of county health services. Even if the communities had been receptive to a new and expanded role, they were not equipped to carry it out. The community groups knew little about physician recruitment or the administrative details associated with establishing a health care center and already were struggling just to organize advisory boards and provide facilities for the centers.

Little progress was made in the ensuing months, and in February 1978, Mr.Tandrell resigned from the hospital to take a position with the state health planning agency. Marvin Sisson, the hospital's director of planning, was assigned Mr. Tandrell's responsibilities for the satellite project. Because of his hospital planning responsibilities, which he viewed as primary, Mr. Sisson spent only about 10 percent of his time on the center project.

In April, Mr. Chapelwaite reversed his earlier decision to give the communities the principal role in the project. There had been no noticeable signs of progress with that approach, and calls from several community leaders with official ties were a key factor in Mr. Chapelwaite's decision to abandon it. In addition to once again taking up the reins, Mr. Chapelwaite directed Mr. Sisson to concentrate all project efforts on opening the Biscoe center, where progress was more advanced. The Warner-Robbins group had already let the lease for the center facility expire after nearly one year without a physician on contract.

Opening the Biscoe Center

With a July 1 target date for opening the Biscoe Center, Dr. Gregerson and Dr. Kistner signed contracts with the hospital in June 1978 *(Exhibit)*. The other positions at the center had been filled for months, but because of the delays in recruiting physicians and opening the center, the nursing assistant and laboratory technician had taken jobs elsewhere. With renovation of the center site under way and the physicians recruited, the community advisory group began making plans to introduce the center and the doctors to the Biscoe community.

The Biscoe center did not open on July 1 because building renovations were not completed. A new target date of August 15th was set. However, a dispute erupted, with Dr. Kistner at odds with the hospital and Dr. Gregerson. Dr. Kistner still refused to participate in the project before the center actually opened, complained that not enough equipment had been purchased for the center and was upset that the target date had been postponed again. Several days before the rescheduled opening of the center, Dr. Kistner obtained legal assistance to extricate himself from the contract.

The Biscoe health center opened in October 1978 with Dr. Gregerson as the physician. Except for the second physician, the center had its full staffing complement as originally planned. Although the center was projected to serve 3,483 patients for a total of 10,450 patient visits by mid-1979, the actual number of patients treated by the end of June 1979 was 1,377, for a total of 3,207 patient visits. The average number of patients treated per hour was three. Dr. Gregerson's style of practice called for a complete patient physical before he would render either episodic or after-hours treatment. The average charge and cost per visit were $13.95 and $39.04, respectively.

Once the center opened, the hospital was only marginally involved in its functioning, and Dr. Gregerson took on the task of recruiting a second physician. In late May, the hospital signed a contract with an Alamance Memorial Hospital family practice resident to begin as the center's second physician on July 1, 1979.

Just as Mr. Chapelwaite was beginning to believe that things had worked out after all, problems emerged. First, he discovered that the Montgomery County Hospital's medical staff was organizing a county medical society. One of its purposes was to recruit physicians to set up private practices in the county. The criteria being established for medical society membership related society membership to hospital medical staff affiliation. Despite the hospital's posture of minimal involvement in the health center, the negative attitude of the medical staff toward the satellite project and the hospital's role in it apparently had not subsided as Mr. Chapelwaite had presumed.

Second, dissatisfaction with the hospital's rural primary care efforts was resurging. Mr. Chapelwaite learned that his medical staff were receiving complaints from people in Biscoe who had been refused emergency treatment at the new health center because they did not fall in the category of health center patients. Dr. Loeffler used this to point out to Mr. Chapelwaite that his original predictions of having to serve as back-up for the health center physicians were coming true. Residents of the Warner-Robbins area began demanding explanations from the hospital administrator for the apparent abandonment of that community's health center and threatened to renew their pressure on the county legislature. Finally, the private funding agency, which had extended the hospital's grant period in view of the project delays, was asking Mr. Chapelwaite the same question about the Warner-Robbins health center. The grant agency also was questioning the Biscoe center's low utilization and the justification for a second physician given the patient load.

It seemed to Mr. Chapelwaite that he faced a potentially explosive situation on several fronts. He began asking himself where things had gone wrong and what could be done to stem this new wave of threats.

Exhibit Hospital Contract with Biscoe Center Physicians

County of Montgomery Agreement	This agreement made between Montgomery County Hospital (hereinafter called "Hospital") and _____, M.D. (hereinafter called "Doctor").
Witnesseth:	For and in consideration of the hereinafter described premises, the parties hereunto agree as follows:
Satellite Health Center	Doctor shall provide services of a duly licensed physician in the Satellite Health Center at Biscoe according to a prearranged schedule developed between Doctor and the Citizen's Advisory Council based upon the needs of the Community. Doctor shall have total control of administration of all phases of the Satellite Health Center with right of overview reserved to the Hospital.
Term	This agreement shall remain in full force and effect for a period of one (1) year from July 1, 1978 unless terminated by ninety (90) days written notice by either party to the other or unless immediately terminated for cause.

Equipment and Supplies	The Hospital shall provide all expendable and nonexpendable drugs, supplies, furniture, fixtures and X-ray equipment which are required for the efficient operation of the Satellite Health Center; Hospital's policy for purchasing goods and services shall apply to the Satellite Health Center.
Personnel	The Hospital shall provide the service of professional and other personnel as may be needed for the efficient operation of the Satellite Health Center. The Doctor, with recommendations from the Project Director, shall perform employee evaluations and make recommendations for continued employment and merit increases. The salaries, benefits, and personnel policies applicable to persons assigned to the Satellite Health Center shall be consistent with those of other employees in similar personnel classifications.
Staff Membership	In accordance with, and subject to the procedures of the organized Medical Staff, Doctor is granted and accepts appointment as a member of the Courtesy Medical Staff. Notwithstanding any other provisions hereof, this agreement shall terminate automatically if the staff privileges of Doctor are revoked for cause upon recommendation of the organized Medical Staff. Likewise Doctor's membership on the Medical Staff shall automatically terminate upon termination of this agreement.
Patient Care	Doctor agrees at all times during the term of this agreement, to make available prompt treatment to persons who come or are brought to the Satellite Health Center in need of such treatment, irrespective of ability to pay. Such treatment shall be of the highest type consistent with the facilities available and the standards established in the medical community of which the Satellite Health Center is a part.
Fees	A schedule of fees will be adopted by the Doctor according to those being reasonable and customary for the community. Doctor agrees to neither make nor collect a fee for services rendered to a patient of the Satellite Health Center, other than that made by the Center.
Medical Records	Doctor shall maintain adequate medical records for all persons treated in the Satellite Health Center on a current basis and shall supply the Hospital with such information on such forms (developed by Doctor) as it may, from time to time, request concerning such records.
Independent Contractor	In performing under this agreement, Doctor shall be at all times acting and performing as an independent contractor. The Hospital shall neither have nor exercise any control or direction over the practice of medicine by the Doctor. The sole interest of the Hospital is to assure that medical services shall be performed in a competent, efficient, and satisfactory manner.

Ethics and Standards	Doctor shall engage in medical practice in the Satellite Health Center in accordance with the ethical and professional standards of the American Medical Association, the American Academy of Family Practice and the standards of the Joint Commission on Accreditation of Hospitals.
Liability Insurance	The Hospital shall provide adequate professional liability insurance for the Doctor, with basic coverage not less than $100,000 per occurrence or $300,000 per aggregate claim, and excess coverage up to $1,000,000. The Hospital or community shall also provide general liability insurance for the physical plant apart from the professional liability insurance.
Compensation	Doctor shall receive an annual salary of Forty-Eight Thousand ($48,000) Dollars payable semimonthly on the first and fifteenth of each month.
Annual Leave	Doctor shall have Fifteen (15) working days per year annual leave from the Satellite Health Center for vacation and Fourteen (14) days per year sick leave.
Professional Leave	Doctor shall have additional professional leave so that doctor can obtain annually a minimum of fifty (50) hours Category I Continuing Medical Education credit. All reasonable expenses related to this leave are at Center's expense.
Other Employment	Doctor agrees to devote the first of his professional efforts to the Satellite Health Center, but shall be permitted to engage in additional private practice on his own provided that the same does not interfere with the performance of his duties under this agreement.
Additional Benefits	Hospital will provide Doctor with adequate family major medical insurance.

In Witness Whereof the parties hereto affix their hands and seals this _____ day of _____,1978.

_____(SEAL)

In the Presence of:

_____

Montgomery County Hospital
(SEAL)

By: _____
    Its President

10
Lakeview Hospital

Lakeview Hospital

In 1975, the W. K. Kellogg Foundation funded a $3.5-million project for demonstrating innovations in ambulatory primary care in medically underserved areas. The Hospital Research and Educational Trust was administrator of the project. One of the ambulatory primary care initiatives funded under this project was sponsored by Lakeview Hospital in Butler County, Iowa. The funding of this site and the others under the project stemmed from four major foundation precepts:

- ☐ "The [Kellogg] Foundation sees a need for hospitals to be more responsive to the communities they serve.

- ☐ Access to health care in underserved areas is a national problem.

- ☐ There are resources in the community that can be used to meet the need for medical care.

- ☐ The Foundation wants to see those community resources being used to provide access to and availability of a stable source of care in underserved areas."

Eastern Butler County, Iowa

The city of Lakeview (population 350,000) occupies the northwest portion of triangular-shaped Butler County *(Figure 1)*. The remainder of the county extends approximately 11 miles to the east of Lakeview's city limits. In 1970, the eastern portion of Butler County had a population of 33,050. Both affluent and extremely poor communities are located within eastern Butler County. The affluent communities, with sizable middle- and upper-income populations, are the suburban communities of Lakeview, while poor communities occupy the remainder of eastern Butler County. The percentage of the population living below the poverty level in eastern Butler County doubled between 1970 and 1978, from 9.5 to 18.1 percent. There are six specific poverty areas located within the eastern portion of the county. Of all these areas, Newton-Perry had the highest percentage of black persons (37.7 percent), persons over 65 (10.5 percent) and persons living below the poverty level (13.2 percent) in 1970.

Eastern Butler County has long been unable to attract sufficient full-time medical practitioners to meet its health care needs. It was

Figure 1 Butler County, Iowa

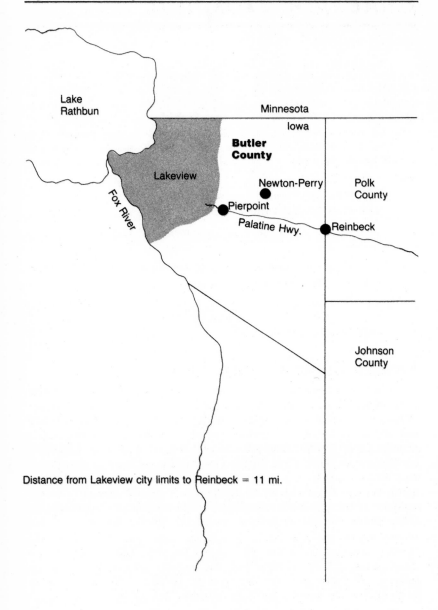

Distance from Lakeview city limits to Reinbeck = 11 mi.

estimated that the needs of its 1970 population could support approximately 17 primary care physicians; in contrast, only five were practicing in the area. Communities at the eastern border of Butler County were 30 minutes by automobile from Lakeview Hospital. In April 1978, portions of eastern Butler County were designated as medically underserved areas.

The director of the State Health Planning and Development Agency gave several reasons for the area's inaccessibility to primary medical care: "Lack of public transportation is the major barrier. In addition, the barriers of socioeconomic status, ethnicity and unwillingness of physicians to accept Medicaid and Medicare patients should be considered. Eastern Butler County is 'artificially' isolated from Lakeview area health resources by the existence of quite affluent residential areas between the City of Lakeview and the rest of the eastern county area."

Health Care Delivery Efforts

The Butler County Health Department has provided preventive health services, primarily in the homes of area clients, since the 1940s. During the 1960s, the department worked with the Office of Economic Opportunity (OEO) and a community advisory group to open a neighborhood health center in Newton-Perry, Newton Township. Despite the community's initial involvement and identification with the center, it closed after three years when federal OEO funding expired. The health department resumed providing only its traditional form of health care—categorical services for specific age or population groups.

In late 1974, Martin Dunlap, M.D., a family practitioner on the staff of Lakeview Hospital, formed the Newton-Perry Medical Corporation, a private practice, to provide free medical services to eastern Butler County's poor. He was joined by Dwight Benne, M.D., another family practitioner who had been chief of staff at Lakeview Hospital since 1973. Drs. Benne and Dunlap set up and financed a practice in which they saw Newton-Perry patients one or two afternoons each week, with a nurse practitioner available four to five days each week. Dr. Dunlap worked closely with the Butler County Health Department, which referred patients to the office.

Dr. Benne later commented that the corporation's original idea had been to obtain physician coverage for the other afternoons. However, because he and Dr. Dunlap were not seeing any private-pay patients at Newton-Perry, they would, in effect, be asking other physicians to donate their time to the care of the area's poor.

Continued operation of the office became a financial burden and the corporation dissolved in March 1976. Dr. Benne believed that Lakeview Hospital should begin providing primary care for the poor residents of eastern Butler County.

Lakeview Hospital

Lakeview Hospital is a 700-bed, private, nonprofit hospital providing secondary and tertiary care to residents of northwestern Iowa. Located in a residential area of Lakeview's east side, the hospital is the largest of the city's six hospitals and provides care to approximately 29,000 patients per year. The hospital has grown substantially in recent years, increasing total revenues from $16 million in 1960 to $90 million in 1970. Jack Schroeder, the hospital's president, explained: "We were a small community hospital that served the area immediately around the institution in 1970 and before that. We are not that way anymore and we will never go back to that."

The hospital is located in what historically was a white, middle-income area of Lakeview. In recent years, the neighborhood's population has become more racially and ethnically diverse, and many whites have moved to the rural and suburban areas surrounding Lakeview. Mr. Schroeder cited the effect of Lakeview's population shifts on Lakeview Hospital: "The middle-income whites are moving into the areas different from where we are located. That is one reason why I think we have to constantly be aware of building a referral base."

The hospital has always had a commitment to the private practice of medicine—supporting the concept of physicians in private practice as opposed to hiring salaried physicians. According to Mr. Schroeder, the hospital had an equally strong commitment to developing hospital-based ambulatory care programs, primarily to find additional sources of referrals. These two commitments are reflected in the L. L. Reiland family practice program which, under the direction of Tyler Cartwright, M.D., of the hospital's medical staff, is affiliated with the Medical College of Iowa and located at Lakeview Hospital. The family practice program trains family practitioners and assists its residents in establishing local practices. As part of its long-range goals for ambulatory care, the hospital planned to build two ambulatory care buildings behind the hospital to house the L. L. Reiland family practice program, several of the hospital's other ambulatory care programs and rental offices for 40 to 60 private physicians.

Proposal for a Lakeview Hospital Ambulatory Care Satellite

When the Newton-Perry Medical Corporation was dissolved in March 1976, Dr. Benne approached Lakeview Hospital's board of trustees and Mr. Schroeder with the idea of opening a hospital-supported satellite physicians' office in the Newton-Perry area. Dr. Benne proposed establishing "a medical center providing family practice care with a personal physician/patient relationship in a clinic situation. It would serve not only the people of the Newton-Perry area who received various types of public assistance, but also the private-pay population in eastern Butler County." Dr. Benne's proposal to include private-pay patients was intended as a financial incentive for the hospital to set up a primary care center that would provide care to the area's poor.

Mr. Schroeder viewed the idea of a hospital-supported satellite from a different perspective—that of expanding the hospital's revenue bases, adding medical staff and building a broader referral base. For the hospital to continue drawing from its present patient group of middle-income whites, it would need to establish a referral base in the eastern suburban areas to which members of this group were moving. He saw the hospital's emphasis on family practice as an important component of that referral system. He and the board opted to establish the center.

During the summer of 1976, Carl Steadham, assistant hospital administrator for corporate planning and budgeting *(Figure 2)*, explored potential public and private funding sources to finance the proposed satellite center. In July 1976, he applied to the Hospital Research and Educational Trust for W. K. Kellogg Foundation funds being offered for ambulatory primary care delivery efforts in under-served areas of the United States.

In the application, Lakeview Hospital proposed opening a health care center in or near Newton-Perry to provide medical services to the medically underserved areas of eastern Butler, western Polk and northwestern Johnson counties. The center would be an outpatient department of the hospital and function within the hospital's policy and procedure structures. The hospital would staff the center with a full-time family practice physician/medical director, as well as an office manager, nurse practitioner, medical assistant and receptionist/housekeeper. It also intended to "utilize all appropriate classifications of nonphysician providers, such as nurse practitioners, clinical pharmacists and clinical psychologists, and to provide services in a facility

244

Figure 2 Lakeview Hospital Organizational Chart (1976)

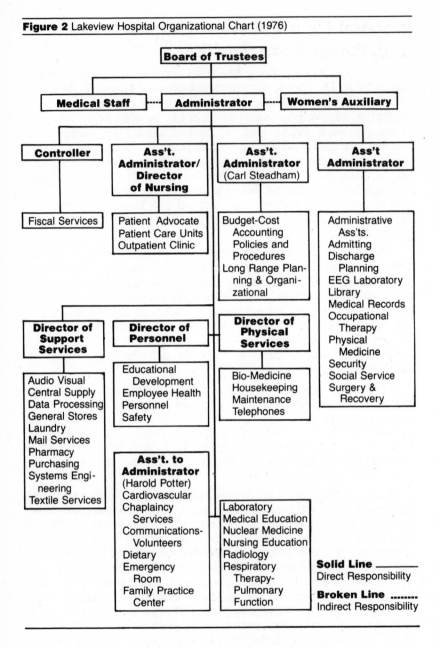

Solid Line _____
Direct Responsibility

Broken Line ....
Indirect Responsibility

that would resemble one of our local physician family practice offices." Proposed services included those offered in any family physician's office, plus laboratory work and minor emergency care. Physical therapy services and patient education programs were slated as third-year initiatives.

Because the center would be an outpatient department of the hospital, its physicians would be members of the hospital medical staff and its employees would be hospital employees. The hospital would perform billing, purchasing and other administrative support functions for the center. Most center patients requiring hospitalization would be referred to Lakeview Hospital. As an outpatient department of the hospital, the center would be governed by the Lakeview Hospital board of trustees. The board would not be involved in the day-to-day operations of the center, but would regularly consider center affairs through its executive committee. Day-to-day decision making would be the responsibility of the center's medical director. The assistant hospital administrator responsible for the center would carefully monitor its operation and provide assistance as needed.

Lakeview Hospital planned to work closely with the Butler County Health Department in marketing the center and its services to residents of the service area. Paula Mathis, R.N., director of nursing for the health department, had worked with Mr. Steadham on the grant proposal. The arrangement between the two parties included a verbal agreement that the health department would help mobilize the residents of Newton-Perry for an informal advisory group for the satellite center.

In response to the hospital's initial grant application in July 1976 *(Figure 3),* the grant agency advised Lakeview Hospital that a favorable review would require clarification and justification of several budget line items, as well as "clearer evidence of significant community involvement" in the project. The hospital revised its application accordingly *(Figure 4),* adding the following reference to community involvement:

> It has been established that an Advisory Board—
> composed of representatives of various local consumer groups representing the service area such as:
> churches and PTAs; welfare departments; and neighborhood opportunity centers—be set up to serve as an advisor to the Lakeview Hospital Family Care Center on health and welfare issues as they relate to the service provided by the Center. The Advisory Board is also to serve as a community forum for the

Figure 3 Lakeview Hospital Budget Projections for Lakeview Family Care Center*
(Submitted in grant application July 1976)

Expenses	Year 1	Year 2	Year 3
Physician(s)	$ 40,000	$ 40,000	$ 40,000
Nurse practitioner(s)	20,000	20,000	20,000
Aide	8,000	8,000	8,000
Business manager	12,000	12,000	12,000
Housekeeper	6,000	6,000	6,000
Subtotal	86,000	86,000	86,000
Finge benefits @ 20%	17,200	17,200	17,200
Total Salaries	103,200	103,200	103,200
Office supplies	2,400	2,400	2,400
Medical supplies	10,000	10,000	10,000
Equipment rental	3,000	3,000	3,000
Other utilities and contingencies	12,400	12,400	12,400
Medical testing	20,000	20,000	20,000
Patient outreach service and transportation	20,000	20,000	20,000
Patient education (preventive care)	24,000	24,000	24,000
Space rental	9,000	9,000	9,000
Total Expenses	100,800	100,800	100,800
Total Operating Expenses	$204,000	$204,000	$204,000
Income			
Patients	$ 6,000	$ 11,000	$ 12,000
Medicare	15,000	26,000	37,000
Medicaid	15,000	26,000	37,000
Blue Shield	12,000	20,000	28,000
Other insurance	6,000	11,000	12,000
Subtotal	54,000	94,000	126,000
†Other	—	—	78,000
Hospital Research and Educational Trust	150,000	110,000	-0-
Total Income	$204,000	$204,000	$204,000
Expected number of patient visits	4,000	6,500	9,400

*Self-sufficiency expected in year four.
†Expected Rural Health Initiative grant.

Figure 4 Lakeview Hospital Revised Budget Projections for Lakeview Family Care Center (Submitted in grant application February 1977)*

Expenses	Year 1	Year 2	Year 3
Physician(s)	$ 40,000	$ 40,000	$ 42,000
Nurse	10,000	10,000	10,500
Aide and housekeeper	8,000	8,000	8,400
Business manager	10,000	12,000	12,600
Subtotal	70,000	70,000	73,500
5% annual increase	-0-	3,500	3,700
Fringe benefits @ 20%	14,000	14,700	15,400
†Contractual services			
Patient education (preventive care)	12,000	-0-	-0-
Patient outreach services and transportation	20,000	10,000	-0-
Total salaries & contractual services	116,000	98,000	92,600
Office supplies	2,400	2,400	2,400
Medical supplies	10,000	10,000	10,000
Equipment rental	3,000	3,000	3,000
‡Utilities & contingencies	12,400	12,400	12,400
Space rental	9,000	9,000	9,000
Subtotal	36,800	36,800	36,800
Total Operating Expenses	$152,800	$135,000	$129,400
Income			
Patients	$ 6,000	$ 9,000	$ 12,000
Medicare	15,000	25,000	39,000
Medicaid	15,000	25,000	39,000
Blue Shield	12,000	18,000	38,000
Other insurance	6,000	9,000	12,000
Subtotal	54,000	86,000	140,000
Hospital Research and Educational Trust	98,800	49,000	-0-
Total Income	$152,800	$135,000	$140,000
Expected number of patient visits	4,000	6,500	9,600

*Financial projections have been revised and reflect reaching self-sufficiency in third year of operation.

†Patient outreach: contracts to be negotiated with existing public health agencies to provide service until year 3 when self-sufficiency should be reached. Patient education: contracts to be negotiated with public agencies to assist in set up and service delivery in year 1; thereafter will be assumed by hospital and health center.

‡With rising costs and inflation, accurate projection impossible for utilities. Contingencies represent the dollar amount of patient accounts estimated to be uncollectible.

resolution of health and welfare issues as they pertain
to the area.

In March 1977, the Hospital Research and Educational Trust
awarded Lakeview Hospital a two-year, $147,000 grant, effective July
1977, to launch the center.

Center Start-Up and Early Growth

Assistant administrator Steadham was assigned responsibility for
setting up the center. In August 1977, he recruited two physicians
from the L. L. Reiland family practice program to staff the center.
Rodney Moore, M.D., began accepting referrals from the service area
at the hospital and Robert Sanchez, M.D., would join the center upon
completion of his residency in July 1978.

Although the hospital planned to open the center on August 1,
1977, problems in securing an adequate building in an appropriate
location delayed its opening. Mr. Schroeder later said that very few
suitable buildings were available for rent in the Newton-Perry area
and building a facility would have been too costly. In September 1977,
the hospital signed a 10-year lease for the first floor of a building on
Palatine Highway in Pierpoint, a Lakeview suburb located in Newton
Township. Although space was limited, additional second-floor space
could be leased later to accommodate the center's planned third-year
programs. The hospital contracted with a local firm to renovate the
facility, and this work further delayed the center's opening.

The Pierpoint location differed from the original plan to locate the
center in Newton-Perry. Pierpoint is 30 minutes east of downtown
Lakeview and approximately four miles from Newton-Perry. Lakeview's population growth to the east and southeast had resulted in
constant expansion down Palatine Highway, a main east-west thor-
oughfare.

Dr. Benne, who had initially proposed that the center serve the
Newton-Perry patients that he and Dr. Dunlap had once served, was
disappointed with the center's location: "It was in a better location to
serve the people of eastern Butler County who were the private-pay
type. It was not really the best location to serve the people of
Newton-Perry." Mr. Schroeder disagreed: "The question, I think,
boils down more to finances than anything else. But finding a place
was limited as to what was available. The grant application, if I
remember correctly, was only to serve the rural area. It didn't identify
with the underprivileged." Dr. Benne also noted that some of the
hospital's medical staff felt that the change in location from Newton-

Perry to Pierpoint put the center in competition with Pierpoint area private physicians for private-pay patients. Mrs. Mathis also was unhappy with the location. She felt that it would be difficult to attract Newton-Perry patients to the center and even more so to involve them in an advisory board.

In October 1977, administration of the center project was transferred from Mr. Steadham to another assistant administrator, Harold Potter, signaling a change from planning to operations. In November 1977, a contractual agreement was signed with the Butler County Health Department whereby the hospital would pay the salary of one full-time health department nurse who would screen health department patients from eastern Butler County for possible referral to the center. Mr. Potter also arranged for the center to access the services of a dietician and clinical psychologist on the staff of the L. L. Reiland family practice program.

The Lakeview Hospital Family Care Center opened on December 1, 1977, staffed by medical director Moore, one nurse and one bookkeeper/receptionist. Mr. Potter reported that the single biggest problem the center experienced during its first month of operation was one of image: "Newspaper articles with misinformation, which ran at the time the hospital announced its intention to establish the center, have created the perception that the family care center is simply a clinic to serve indigent patients. The center was established to help meet the medical needs of the indigent, but also to develop a patient population which could fully support the operation of the center within three years."

In February 1978, Mr. Potter began addressing community organizations to encourage local understanding and utilization of the center. He had articles about the center published in local papers, put local leaders on the hospital's mailing list and held a center open house in March. Dr. Moore also joined the marketing/promotion effort by speaking to local community groups. Both Mr. Potter and the center staff believed that word of mouth was the most effective tool for promoting the center.

After a slow start, the center's utilization levels for the first six months of operation (December 1977 through May 1978) indicated steady growth, with a total of 311 new patients and 956 patient visits. During that period, self-pay patients accounted for 75 percent of the center's gross billings, Medicare and Medicaid patients each comprised 10 percent and Blue Cross patients constituted 5 percent. Most patients were under 30 years of age. The figures indicated that many residents of Reinbeck, a middle-income farming community nine miles east of the health center, were utilizing center services.

In July 1978, the hospital began discussions with the University of Lakeview's graduate program in community health education to develop a questionnaire to identify and measure the health needs of the eastern Butler County population. This project was postponed by Lakeview Hospital.

Community Advisory Board for the Center

Although the formation of a community advisory board had been planned, no board had been formed by April 1978. Mrs. Mathis reported difficulty in recruiting Newton-Perry community members. "The patients our nurses referred to the center were reluctant to go there for care and even more reluctant to return for follow-up visits. Patients reported feeling uncomfortable in the office, partly because Pierpoint wasn't their community." Mr. Potter had spoken to several local Rotary clubs about forming a Pierpoint-based advisory group, but was not successful. He requested information from the grant agency on the formation, purpose and responsibilities of community advisory boards.

In a July 1978 meeting with grant agency staff, Mr. Potter questioned the usefulness of a community advisory board for the center given the nature of the hospital/center/community relationship. He alluded to four problem areas:

☐ The center was a department of the hospital and under the jurisdiction of the hospital's board—an arrangement limiting the possible role of a community advisory board.

☐ It would be difficult to form a representative board for the center because the communities within its service area ranged from depressed rural areas to fairly prosperous suburbs.

☐ The low-income residents in the community were negative about advisory boards because of the earlier failure of the local OEO clinic, which had a community advisory board.

☐ Advisory boards with no real decision-making powers tended to be short-lived.

Second-Year Growth

The center recorded 6,396 patient visits for the year ending June 30, 1979. Over 40 percent of the patients were from Pierpoint and Reinbeck. Patient profiles showed that 29 percent of the patients served were 15 years of age or younger. The percentage of the center's gross billings generated by private-pay patients had risen from the 75 percent reported in its first six months of operation to 89.6 percent, while the share of Medicare and Medicaid billings had dropped from 10 percent each to 6.4 percent and 0.5 percent respectively. After 18 months of operation, the center was close to financial self-sufficiency —a goal the hospital expected the center to reach by September 1979.

Although the center had been established in an area outside the boundaries of any organized community, by July 1978 the center had succeeded in initiating a relationship with the Reinbeck area Chamber of Commerce—a relationship based on the increasing number of Reinbeck residents using the center—that helped to identify the center with a particular community. According to Mr. Potter, "Community involvement is helpful but not essential for success of the type of program that we have established at the family care center."

Changes in Staffing

Mr. Potter left his position in August 1979. Following his departure, the hospital combined responsibility for all ambulatory care activities under one individual who could concentrate on ambulatory care without the distractions of many other responsibilities. In November 1979, the hospital hired health care management consultant Christopher Tannenbaum and assigned him responsibility for all ambulatory care programs *(Figure 5)*.

Proposal for Patient and Community Health Education Programs

Based on nearly two years of center growth, the hospital wanted to expand the Pierpoint center programs beyond medical services to include the health education programs originally planned as third-year activities. In October 1979, the hospital submitted a proposal to the Hospital Research and Educational Trust for supplemental third-year funding to implement a patient health education program at the center, followed by a community health education program. The long-term aim of the programs, according to the proposal, was to reduce demand for costly acute medical services by teaching people to be responsible for their own health.

For the patient education program—phase 1 of the hospital's plan—patient screening and referrals would be handled by the center physicians. Professional staff from Lakeview Hospital and the L. L. Reiland family practice program then would visit the center on a scheduled basis to provide education services to the patients referred. The community health education program—phase 2 of the plan—

Figure 5 Lakeview Hospital Organizational Chart (Effective 11-79)

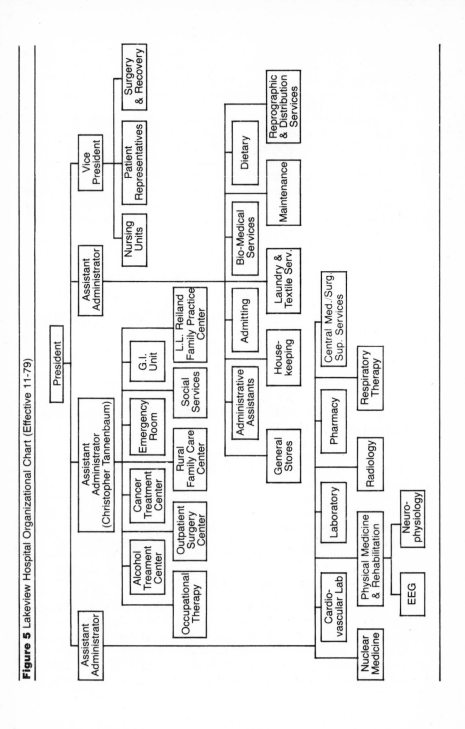

represented a more ambitious undertaking. This program would be conducted in group settings for community members interested in health maintenance. The hospital selected weight loss, nutrition, breast self-examination, stress reduction and smoking cessation clinics for the phase 2 program. The selection was based on 1976 Butler County mortality data on the five leading causes of death—data that coincided with national norms.

According to the hospital's proposal, "Patient education has been a secondary goal of the family care center after growth and self-sufficiency are realized." The hospital saw the education programs as a means of increasing center utilization and, in turn, increasing the hospital's potential referral base.

The person on the hospital staff who wrote the grant proposal for the supplemental funding was Walter Carey, recently appointed to the new position of director of grants after serving as the hospital's administrative services coordinator. Mr. Carey saw the education programs from yet another perspective. His interest was in using the Pierpoint center education programs as a pilot. If successful, the pilot project would form the basis for receiving additional grant funds to develop a health education package that could be sold to other clinics, outreach centers or hospitals that could use that type of program.

The hospital planned to hire a patient education coordinator to administer the program. Dr. Cartwright, director of the family practice program, and his staff would provide practical direction and support for the programs as well as aid center staff through consultative services for patients. For some time, Dr. Cartwright had been working closely with the hospital's Education Department to develop programs for the L. L. Reiland family practice program similar to those planned for the center. The Education Department would participate in decisions regarding the content and process for the center's five community health programs.

Lakeview Hospital's application for supplemental funding for the health education activities was returned because of major discrepancies between budget projections and program objectives. The hospital was advised to reassess the cost versus benefits stated in the proposal and justify program self-sufficiency after grant support ended. Another problem was the absence of a community advisory mechanism for the community health education plans. Once again, the hospital revised its initial proposal at the grant agency's urging *(Figures 6 and 7)*. The Reinbeck Chamber of Commerce's interest in the center was reflected in the hospital's revised funding application:

Figure 6 Lakeview Hospital Expenditure Summary Lakeview Family Care Center (Submitted in supplemental grant application October 1979)

Category	Total Health Center	Health Education Programs (Requested from Hospital Research and Educational Trust)
Salaries	$154,150	$25,860
Fringe benefits	38,537	6,465
Consultants	4,800	4,800
Travel	1,500	-0-
Medical supplies	13,086	-0-
Office supplies	13,161	10,661
Space rental	18,936	8,100
Utilities	9,200	2,000
Maintenance	1,620	-0-
Printing and subscription	1,500	500
Telephone	1,800	-0-
Program faculty	9,118	9,118
Total Direct Expense	**$267,408**	**$67,504**

Figure 7 Lakeview Hospital Expenditure Summary Lakeview Family Care Center (Submitted in supplemental grant application November 1979)

Category	Total Health Center	Health Education Programs (Requested from Hospital Research and Educational Trust)
Salaries	$150,250	$21,960
Fringe benefits	37,562	5,490
Consultants	4,800	4,800
Travel	2,500	1,000
Medical supplies	13,086	-0-
Office supplies	13,161	1,342
*Space rental	18,936	2,760
†Utilities	9,200	1,000
Maintenance	1,620	-0-
Printing and subscription	2,000	1,000
Telephone	1,800	300
Program faculty	9,118	9,118
Total Direct Expense	**$264,033**	**$48,760**

*The available space at the Lakeview Family Care Center does not permit use of the facility for the group education activities proposed. Space rental cost suitable for these activities will run approximately $3.00 per square foot per annum; this portion of the proposal will require 920 square feet.

†The present rate in the area for utilities is slightly above $1.00 per square foot per annum.

In working with the Reinbeck, Iowa, Chamber of Commerce, we have established the foundation of a community advisory committee. We feel strongly that existing community leaders should take the lead in identifying and organizing a community advisory group. The Reinbeck Chamber of Commerce has agreed to take the lead and involve people in the community with the establishment of the proposed health education programs.

According to the application, the patient education coordinator and Mr. Tannenbaum would meet with the Reinbeck Chamber of Commerce leaders during December 1979. Monthly meetings with the community advisory board appointed by the Chamber of Commerce would begin during January 1980. During February 1980, the advisory board would formulate policies on expanding the patient education programs to community education programs.

In November 1979, the Hospital Research and Educational Trust awarded Lakeview Hospital supplemental funding of $48,760 to support educational programming at the center from December 1, 1979, through November 30, 1980. The patient and community education programs were to be financially self-sufficient by the end of the funding period.

Implementing the Health Education Programs

Charity Hawkins, a health educator at Lakeview Hospital responsible for in-service education programs, was appointed the center's patient education coordinator in February 1980, three months into the grant period. Her charge included establishing a community advisory board for the community health program, determining the appropriate combination of educational modalities and coordinating the programs.

Mrs. Hawkins' position was viewed by the hospital as a cooperative effort between the hospital and the center. She reported to assistant administrator Tannenbaum and her contact at the center for the education programs was Dr. Sanchez. She retained her office at the hospital due to space limitations at the center. Mrs. Hawkins attempted to spend several days each week at the center, but found that her work developing the programs kept her at the hospital more than anticipated.

Mrs. Hawkins' first two months as patient education coordinator were spent primarily on locating a facility in which to conduct the center's education programs. The hospital planned to conduct the community health education program in public buildings because of space limitations at the center. The original plan to rent additional space on the second floor of the center building was abandoned because of the cost and poor access (the building had no elevators). Mrs. Hawkins finally decided to lease and furnish a trailer near the center for office and instruction space. The trailer would be used for the patient education sessions and for the smaller community education clinics that did not require the amount of space available in public buildings.

The patient education program was implemented with ease because it required only that Mrs. Hawkins schedule hospital staff according to the service needs of specific patient groups. The community education program required that Mrs. Hawkins design the five programs selected, set up a scheduling system for referrals by area physicians, work with the hospital's Marketing Department to publicize the programs and work with the hospital's Media Services Department to design motivational posters and informational literature. She expected to implement at least four and possibly all five of the programs by April 1, 1980.

The education programs being designed by Mrs. Hawkins were not being met with open arms by the center's physicians. Dr. Moore, the medical director, said: "We want to run this as a private doctors' office. We want to take care of our own patients. It is the only way to keep them satisfied. . . . This [center] is different than a private practice, but works basically that way. It is different because of the hospital involvement."

Mrs. Hawkins had hoped to meet with Drs. Moore and Sanchez on a weekly basis to work out the details of the project, but had difficulty getting them to agree to regularly scheduled meetings. Both physicians recognized the value of health education but were reluctant to incorporate the hospital-developed programs into their practices. Dr. Moore already had incorporated similar efforts, such as hypertension education and breast self-examination, into his practice. He preferred these efforts to the new community education program, which he said "is taking too long to develop. It is too large to do practically. The practice is not large enough to support the program as it is conceived and planned."

At about this time, when final plans were being made for the community health education programs, Mr. Carey met with the grant agency staff to present a proposal for altering the original plans. The hospital wanted to separate the community education programs from the health center and conduct them under the sponsorship of the L. L. Reiland family practice program. The grant agency declined to approve the request and threatened to withdraw the supplemental funding if the hospital did not adhere to the intent of the original application.

Community Advisory Board for the Education Programs

Development of the education programming was well under way, but no attempt had been made to establish a community advisory board. Mr. Tannenbaum felt that an advisory board was not necessary to the project's success. He had worked with advisory groups at a California hospital and found that their meetings tended to be complaint sessions that generated little or no help in planning or decision making. He said, "We could do health education programming equally as well without an advisory group. Advisory groups are more trouble than they're worth."

Mr. Tannenbaum felt that the Lakeview Hospital board of trustees and executive committee provided the best direction and policy formation for the center. However, both he and Mrs. Hawkins agreed that an advisory board could be used as a marketing tool for the programs. Mrs. Hawkins renewed the center's relationship with the Reinbeck Chamber of Commerce by arranging an April 1980 meeting with Mr. Hunt, the chamber's president, to discuss the formation of a community advisory board.

The five community education programs were scheduled to begin on April 30, 1980, and Drs. Moore and Sanchez were already generating referrals to them when Mrs. Hawkins met with Mr. Hunt at the beginning of April. Following that initial meeting, Mr. Hunt invited Mrs. Hawkins and Mr. Tannenbaum to a formal chamber meeting to discuss the plans for community education programming. Chamber members were enthusiastic about the programs but unaware that they already had been developed and scheduled. Mr. Hunt and the chamber members suggested assessing community needs and interests in different programs and hours, adding an exercise class and beginning with one or two programs instead of all five.

During the month of May, the center introduced its programs as scheduled.

11
Cape Meares Health Clinic

Cape Meares Health Clinic

In the summer of 1976, Angela Traynor, administrator and sole provider for the Cape Meares Health Clinic, received approval from the clinic's board of directors to apply for a grant being offered by the Hospital Research and Educational Trust. The clinic was awarded $115,000 for a two-year period, effective January 1, 1977. Mrs. Traynor wanted to use the funds to expand the clinic's hours of operation from two to five days a week, to increase staff and to initiate outreach services and health promotion programs *(see Exhibit)*. What Mrs. Traynor did not foresee was that the grant also would provoke a change in the clinic board's composition, size, leadership and level of involvement in clinic affairs. Over the next two years, Mrs. Traynor and the new board president, Roy Eldridge, would struggle bitterly and often over such issues as clinic utilization, finances, staffing and community image.

Founding of Cape Meares Health Clinic

Angela Traynor maintained a farm near Fayetteville, Oregon, and was active in the small Cape Meares community. She had earned a reputation as a caring, people-oriented and committed nursing professional. Most of her nursing experience had been with small, nonprofit operations, and she often commented that she felt most comfortable and effective when engaged in community service. Her experience also included three years as director of nursing services for a nursing home.

In the 30 years Mrs. Traynor had practiced nursing in and around Portland and Tillamook County, she had developed good contacts with other local health care providers and an understanding of the health care needs of Cape Meares' predominantly rural and low-income population. In 1972, she began an active and successful campaign to establish primary care services for the cape, principally for its poor. With no physicians on the cape, the 2,900 permanent and 3,000 summer residents who needed medical care traveled to Tillamook or Portland *(Figure 1)*. When the federal government designated the cape as a medically underserved area in early 1978, it was largely the result of Mrs. Traynor's efforts.

Figure 1 Tillamook County, Oregon

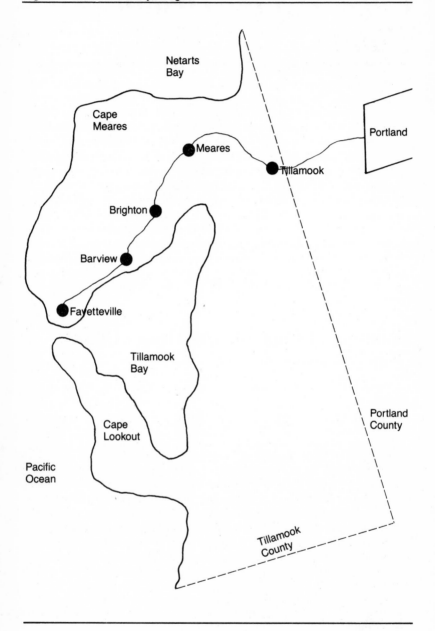

Netarts
Bay

Cape
Meares

Portland

Meares

Tillamook

Brighton

Barview

Fayetteville

Tillamook
Bay

Portland
County

Cape
Lookout

Pacific
Ocean

Tillamook
County

With the help of community donations of money, time and a converted beach house for the facility, Mrs. Traynor established the Cape Meares Health Clinic in Fayetteville as a nonprofit corporation. The service area was intended to encompass all of Cape Meares and nearby Cape Lookout although concentrating on the Fayetteville area.

The clinic was set up primarily to serve the indigent, whom Mrs. Traynor felt were most in need of affordable and accessible basic medical care. By volunteering her services and getting other community people to do likewise, Mrs. Traynor operated the clinic two days a week, asking patients to pay for the services only to the extent they were able. Many received care at no cost. Mrs. Traynor stated: "When I set this clinic up, I felt that the cape's poor should have equal access to health care services. I saw the clinic as serving this special population, and doing so was a gesture of good will by the larger community. I never expected the original clinic to generate any income, but when it began to in 1975, I thought that the medical need on the cape went beyond the poor.* So I started looking around for a way to expand the services to more people and saw that the Hospital Research and Educational Trust grant would serve that purpose."

By January 1, 1977, the Cape Meares Health Clinic had been operating four years, providing services two days a week. Some of the services were provided cooperatively by the clinic and other area health care organizations, such as the county health department.

Clinic Staffing

Mrs. Traynor received minimal compensation for her services as the clinic's director and nurse practitioner. During the two days a week the clinic was open, she devoted her time to patient care and spent an additional two days a week on administrative duties. The clinic was staffed almost entirely by volunteers from the community. Mrs. Traynor started out in 1972 with two volunteer registered nurses, who also were on the board, and a paid receptionist. By 1976, a third R.N., a bookkeeper and a laboratory technician had been added to the volunteer staffing complement. At Mrs. Traynor's request, the county medical society appointed two physician preceptors from Portland who performed periodic medical audits, provided consultation services and served as referral physicians for clinic patients. They volunteered those services until the clinic was able to provide an annual stipend from the grant funds.

Upon receipt of the grant funds, Mrs. Traynor set out to expand

---

*By mid-1976, clinic income averaged $600 per month and patients treated averaged over 140 per month.

the staffing complement by adding full-time health professionals. In June 1977, she hired a nurse practitioner, Shirley Cascade, and an outreach social worker, Lars Taggart. By that point, the clinic was providing services four days a week with Mrs. Traynor continuing in the dual role of nurse practitioner and director at an annual salary of $12,000.

Soon after hiring the new staff, Mrs. Traynor noticed mounting tension between the volunteer and paid staff. When the paid staff took what the volunteers perceived as liberties, such as arriving late for work or taking long breaks, the volunteers often took it upon themselves to reprimand the staff. Mrs. Traynor said, "I realized something had to be done about defining the roles of volunteer and paid staff. But the volunteers had been with the clinic for so long and really were what this clinic is all about. I didn't want to hurt their feelings and have them leave." When Mrs. Traynor began to notice that the volunteers were reporting clinic activities to other board members or at board meetings, however, she decided to act. In late 1978, she developed formal role descriptions for clinic volunteers.

Four months after she was hired as nurse practitioner, Miss Cascade resigned.* Mr. Taggart resigned in December 1978. Meanwhile, Mrs. Traynor continued to rely heavily on her volunteer nurses to provide clinic services.

Referring to the resignations of Shirley Cascade and Lars Taggart, Mrs. Traynor said:

> I was sorry to lose Shirley; she was a good practition-er. I really fault the board for her resignation. She came to me in tears several times, saying that she had received phone calls from board members chastising her about her personal lifestyle. She finally couldn't take it anymore and left. Her official reason was geographic location.
>
> On the other hand, it was good riddance to Lars Taggart. He was young and inexperienced, and while I devoted a lot of time and energy to getting him started, he just couldn't seem to make it. He kept sending clients to Portland and that wasn't helping our finances. I certainly didn't feel that I could trust him—he was carrying information and reports to Roy Eldridge behind my back and I'd get into trouble at board meetings because of it. He wanted to run the

---

*The position remained vacant until utilization levels justified filling it and recruitment efforts were successful, which was March 1978.

clinic but he couldn't even do his own job. I wanted to fire him long ago, but the personnel policies weren't strong enough.

Roy Eldridge recalled his relationship with Mr. Taggart differently:

I did ask Lars to lunch, as I did all new staff members, but we chatted about a lot of things. As time passed, Lars took advantage of my interest by coming to me on two or three occasions to complain about the way Angela was treating him and running the clinic. I reminded him that, although I believed in staff having access to board members, Angela was his superior and I had no intention of intervening. I told him that if he felt strongly enough he was perfectly free to make a formal complaint to the board personnel committee, which he never did.

At one point, Lars told me that he had given Angela a report describing his position and role. The board never saw this report so I asked Angela for it at a board meeting. We never did see the report. It was obvious that Angela and Lars did not get along and in a way I was relieved when financial considerations made it necessary to eliminate his job.

As far as Shirley is concerned, I heard rumors from other board members that Angela and Shirley did not get along—that Angela wanted Shirley to be just like her as far as service delivery went.

Mr. Taggart described his relationship with Mrs. Traynor as volatile. He said that he had tried to become more involved in clinic affairs and even offered to serve as Mrs. Traynor's administrative assistant. He said that, in return, she was suspicious of his motives and left three-page notes around the office referring to his poor performance and unprofessional conduct. He had wanted to leave the clinic long before December 1978, but was unable to find a challenging job.

Utilization and Finances

When the new board took over in May 1977—the fifth month following receipt of the grant—the clinic's utilization and revenue levels were far below projections. By the end of 1977, data showed that utilization and revenue continued at levels insufficient to put the clinic on a course of financial self-sufficiency *(Figures 2 and 3)*. The

Figure 2 Utilization by Month–1/1/77-12/31/78

	New Patients	Patient Visits to Nurse Practitioner	Patient Visits to Social Worker
January '77	22	130	—
February	33	153	—
March	28	166	—
April	45	276	—
May	35	320	—
June	41	252	—
July	44	193	12
August	48	162	19
September	35	131	24
October	58	409	20
November	32	285	26
December	42	262	18
Total Year 1	463	2,739	119
January '78	26	184	36
February	43	198	26
March	57	293	30
April	34	241	27
May	62	261	28
June	39	227	32
July	55	202	24
August	55	230	25
September	69	280	31
October	27	339	31
November	48	146	20
December	38	205	10
Total Year 2	553	2,806	320

number of patients served for the year averaged 228 a month, which was 35 percent below initial projections. The clinic's net revenue from patients for the year represented only 18.5 percent of total operating expenses. The first six months of 1978 were no better for the clinic. The grant would expire on December 31, 1978, yet the clinic's utilization and revenue figures showed little evidence that the clinic would be able to remain open.

Mrs. Traynor described a series of steps she had taken to increase utilization, among them generating local publicity on the clinic, providing outreach social work services and searching for ways to certify the clinic for Medicare participation to better serve the 22 percent of the population over the age of 65. (Under the Rural Health Clinic Services Act of 1977, the clinic became certified for Medicare participation in early 1978.) Mrs. Traynor actually felt, however, that

Figure 3 Statement of Income and Expenses

Income	Year 1 1/1/77-12/31/77	Year 2 1/1/78-12/31/78	Year 3 1/1/79-12/31/79*
Gross Revenues			
Self-pay	$14,147	$15,619	$36,000
Medicare	-0-	3,499	10,000
Medicaid	4,523	6,808	8,000
Private insurers	1,840	3,943	5,000
Total Gross	$20,510	$29,869	$59,000
Net Revenues			
Self-pay	$ 6,917	$14,529	$32,400
Medicare	-0-	2,835	8,100
Medicaid	3,205	5,583	6,560
Private insurers	1,001	1,895	2,350
Total Net	$11,123	$24,842	$49,410
Other Income			
HRET + Interest	$50,088	$56,643	$ -0-
CETA	4,063	-0-	-0-
Donations	1,402	2,338	3,252
Funds to be determined	-0-	-0-	4,758
Total Other	$55,553	$58,981	$ 8,510
Total Income	$66,676	$83,823	$57,420
Expenses			
Personnel			
Physicians	$ 2,400	$ 4,500	3,600
†Nurse practitioners	5,417	13,078	15,120
Director	12,000	16,500	10,000
Social worker	6,427	14,640	1,000‡
Laboratory technician	5,106	6,681	9,000§
Secretary/Receptionist	4,063	5,474	-0-
Fringe benefits	3,874	6,855	5,500
Total Personnel	$39,287	$67,728	$44,220
Non-personnel			
Equipment	$13,195	$ 1,078	$ 1,000
Office supplies	735	1,267	900
Medical supplies	3,043	2,013	2,300
Rent and utilities	1,757	2,340	2,200
Travel	486	857	1,500
Other	1,561	6,164	4,300
Total Non-personnel	$20,777	$13,719	$13,200
Total Expenses	$60,064	$81,447	$57,420

*Projected figures based on December 7, 1978, clinic reorganization.
†Includes fees for back-up nurse practitioners.
‡Contracted service.
§Combined receptionist/laboratory technician position.

the poor utilization was due to a number of factors beyond her control, most of them related to the board or its actions.

One of the factors she cited was the board's decision to establish a sliding fee schedule for patients soon after the grant was awarded. Mrs. Traynor explained, "The board couldn't see why this upset the community members. Local residents had contributed a lot of time and money to see this clinic succeed and now—after the grant money appeared—they were expected to pay every time they walked in the door." Mrs. Traynor viewed the board's decision to establish a fee structure as an attempt to alter the patient mix and discourage the poor from using the clinic.

A second factor Mrs. Traynor cited was that not all the board members utilized the clinic. She viewed that as an impediment to the clinic's image and community acceptance and was angry about it as well.

Finally, Mrs. Traynor pointed to the cancellation of two service expansion plans for financial reasons—the purchase of a van or a car for outreach services and a boat for serving Cape Lookout. Although Mrs. Traynor recognized that the decision was necessary, she also thought it affected the clinic's ability to increase utilization.

Roy Eldridge and others on the board had a different view of the causes for the clinic's utilization and financial picture. According to Mr. Eldridge, "Angela catered to the down-and-out elements of the community; she felt very motherly toward them. The more conventional elements of the community saw the clinic as a 'hippie-haven' and were reluctant to use it. The board recognized that the image had to be changed if the clinic were to succeed on its own."

Another barrier to utilization cited by board members was the lack of patient privacy. The clinic's layout and sound-proofing were not conducive to privacy, and clinic workers had a reputation of not honoring the confidentiality of patient treatment data.

Some members of the board also believed the clinic was in the wrong location to attract patients, an opinion that Mrs. Traynor did not share. The clinic was in Fayetteville for two reasons: Mrs. Traynor's selection of it as the site and the donation of a facility there. However, recent population growth and new construction were taking place further up the cape near Meares. The pin map Mrs. Traynor maintained to identify the clinic's patient sources showed that most patients were from Fayetteville and Barview with a fairly heavy cluster originating from Meares. According to Mr. Eldridge, the board's feelings about the clinic location were based on guesses because of the quality of administrative recordkeeping and reporting to the board. It was not until November 1978 that the board directed Mrs. Traynor to maintain and submit monthly statistical reports identifying patients' geographic origin, sex, age, number of dependents, categories of treatment and method of payment.

In late August 1978, the executive committee of the board sent Mrs. Traynor the following memorandum:

> At our meeting this morning we agreed that our financial situation is very serious and demands urgent action. With your agreement the Committee requested that by September 12, or earlier if possible, you present to us a budget for the final quarter of 1978 based on such grant monies as are presently available plus the total of our net collections for June, July and August, on the assumption that they will be at least equalled during the last quarter. You will also present by at least December 15 another budget for the first quarter of 1979 on the same basis, that is, net collections for September, October, and November plus whatever additional financial resources we have firmly committed at the time. Both budgets should, of course, be constructed so that timely, dignified, fair and orderly measures can be taken to carry out such reduction of services and personnel as may prove necessary.
>
> It is contemplated that the last quarter 1978 budget will be presented to the board for consideration at the regular meeting on October 5.

The Board of Directors

When the Cape Meares Health Clinic corporation and board were formed in 1972, the initial board of eight adopted bylaws that set board size at 8 to 20, with two-year terms of office for directors and a one-year term for the president. Mrs. Traynor was an ex officio member of the board. Initially, the board consisted primarily of Mrs. Traynor's acquaintances and the clinic volunteers and typically experienced high turnover and vacancies that often were not promptly filled. Few of the board members were knowledgeable about health care delivery or experienced in the operation of a nonprofit organization.

During the first four years, the board operated informally, leaving the provision of services, the direction of the clinic and policy decisions to Mrs. Traynor. The activities of the board consisted of volunteering as staff for the clinic where possible, helping revamp and repair the building, organizing fund-raising events such as rummage sales and spaghetti dinners, and canvassing for funds. The board did not meet regularly, did not use standard parliamentary procedure and had only one committee, an executive committee. The bylaws defined the committee as "the officers, immediate past president and such persons as designated by this committee, subject in all respects to the authority and discretion of the board of directors, and between its meetings the executive committee shall have and exercise the power and authority of the board of directors in the management of keeping up the health clinic."

Annual elections for directors of the board were scheduled for May 1977, five months after the clinic received the grant. By this time, Mrs. Traynor had already detected a change in the board, which she attributed to the grant money. She stated: "All of a sudden, I felt much more restricted in operating the clinic. The board was taking on a new level of interest and concern, like imposing a fee schedule for patients and making decisions about the service expansions outlined in the grant proposal. They didn't want me to operate the way I had before but they weren't exactly sure how they did want me to operate. I really think they were scared of all that money and felt uncomfortable with the responsibility."

A New Look for the Board

One position scheduled to be filled at the May 1977 board elections was that of board president, since the incumbent, a volunteer nurse at the clinic, was completing her term of office. On the board at the time was Roy Eldridge, who for almost a year had been occupying the directorship vacated on his wife's death. Mr. Eldridge was a foreign service officer and former ambassador who had moved to Cape Meares in 1970 when he retired. Mr. Eldridge was elected the new president.

In speaking of his election, Mr. Eldridge explained:

> Sometime in March or April I was approached by a member of the executive committee who said the new president had to be someone who would 'stand up to Angela' and, as they thought I might be willing to do so, asked if I would accept the nomination. I said I wanted to talk to Angela first to form an opinion on whether we could work together harmoniously. My conversation with her was inconclusive. Typically, she evaded making any definite statements. I found that it was almost impossible to get her to state her opinion clearly when she had doubts about or was opposed to any proposal. But she did give me enough positive reaction to persuade me to assent to the committee member's proposal.

Mrs. Traynor had mixed feelings about Mr. Eldridge's election. She remarked: "Roy had really pitched in to fill his wife's term, but I believed there were others who had been on the board and members of the community longer than Roy Eldridge who ought to have had the chance to run things." She also said, "I'm just not sure that I completely trust Roy—he thinks he knows a lot about how to run things because of his experience, but this is just a small, simple community with a lot of people who need to be taken care of."

The May board meeting also resulted in the election of nine new members, bringing the board up to its maximum size of 20 (11 men and 9 women). The board members continued to be community residents from various walks of life who were largely unfamiliar with health care delivery, the operation of a nonprofit organization and the role of a board of directors.

One of the new president's first acts was to appoint an *ad hoc* committee to incorporate a board committee structure into the bylaws. The revised bylaws, which were adopted by the 13 board members present on October 16, 1977, created seven new committees: personnel, transportation, nominating, bylaws, community participation/fund raising, public relations and financial and clinical services.

Not all of the board members were satisfied with this new committee structure. One commented: "The committees didn't know what they were supposed to do. There was a transportation committee, but we really didn't have a problem with that. The financial and clinical services committee had no real purpose, and neither did the building committee, which I was on. We didn't really know what role we were supposed to play."

Board / Administrator Relationships

The first of several confrontations between the clinic director and the board took place shortly after the May board meeting when Mrs. Traynor realized that, under the bylaws, the officers should have been elected by the "new board." Since the new board members had not attended the meeting, they had not participated in the election of the officers. Mrs. Traynor contacted one of the board members with this news. Such a furor was generated over it that, after an executive committee discussion of the matter, Mr. Eldridge stated he felt obliged to call a special board meeting. At this special meeting on June 14, all newly elected officers were confirmed by the new board.

Another confrontation stemmed from Mrs. Traynor's displeasure at two tactics she suspected were being used by the executive committee—making decisions on behalf of the board and meeting without her knowledge or participation. She felt that these "secret" meetings reflected a lack of confidence in her abilities and she offered to resign: "I confronted Roy with this and he denied that secret meetings were being held. He said that the board had the utmost confidence in me and the last thing they wanted me to do was resign. So I let it drop but was not convinced that the secret meetings ended."

Mr. Eldridge believed that Mrs. Traynor's feelings about the executive committee were unfounded: "In the period before I became president, the executive committee probably held occasional meetings to which she was not invited. I did inaugurate regular weekly executive committee meetings to which all board members were invited but only a few attended. The size and composition of the board at that time made it an impractical forum for constructive grappling with the problems facing us. I made a point, however, of always having Angela present except on the few occasions—certainly less than 10 percent of the time—when she was on leave or otherwise unable to attend."

At least one board member supported Mrs. Traynor's contention that the executive committee was acting in place of the board: "The board was very large . . . they really just came and sat. Oftentimes there wasn't a quorum. The officers met every week or so and made decisions for the board without letting the board know until after the fact."

Another frustration facing Mrs. Traynor was what she described as board meddling in matters that were her responsibility as clinic director. As one example, she cited an incident that occurred in the summer of 1978 while Mr. Eldridge was on vacation. When someone in the area was bitten by a wild animal, the health department asked Mrs. Traynor whether she would administer rabies vaccine and then called the clinic's physician preceptor, who gave his approval. When Mr. Eldridge returned, he heard of this incident indirectly from a clinic volunteer and met with Mrs. Traynor to question her decision to provide the service. Mrs. Traynor felt that this called her professional competence into question and reflected an improper role for the board.

Some of the board members agreed with Mrs. Traynor's impression that the board was usurping her role. As one member commented, "We found ourselves trying to get involved in a lot of things that should have been the director's role—how the employees were being used and whether they were doing a good job. Those kinds of things were the job of the director. To tell the truth, I'm still not clear on what our role should have been." Another said, "The board did too much running of the clinic, and Eldridge had a talent for getting things his own way."

Other members of the board, however, described Mrs. Traynor as authoritarian and unwilling to let the board tackle policy decisions. They acknowledged her dedication to the clinic and to helping others but faulted her business acumen. One board member commented that she had the enthusiasm and energy to make the clinic succeed and only wanted the board as a symbol of community support. Another said, "I never felt we were getting accurate information. For example, we wanted to know what kinds of diseases were being treated but she didn't want to give us the information." Mr. Eldridge described Mrs. Traynor as "a great provider—sympathetic and perceptive. Her problem was that she thought she was a good administrator."

The label "authoritarian" was applied to Mr. Eldridge as well by some board members. Mr. Eldridge acknowledged that he ran the board in that way and that it caused some resentment, but said he saw no alternative given the decisions that had to be made.

Clinic Reorganization

The budget data prepared by the clinic director in compliance with the August 1978 executive committee memorandum indicated that the clinic was not financially prepared for the expiration of the grant. To sustain operations in 1979, the clinic would need to double revenue from patients in addition to obtaining $36,000 from unidentified "other" sources. The executive committee decided that one way to prepare for 1979 was to reduce expenses by consolidating several staff positions *(Figure 3)*.

On December 7, 1978, the board approved a new clinic staffing pattern and corresponding job descriptions as recommended by the executive committee. A business manager position was created to work in tandem with a clinical services director/nurse practitioner. The laboratory technologist and receptionist/billing clerk positions were combined. The social worker position, vacated with Mr. Taggart's resignation during this month, was left unfilled until funding became available. The clinic retained the positions of a federally funded 20-hour-per-week office aide and a full-time nurse practitioner, the latter position held by Jack Cicero since March 1978.

Mrs. Traynor agreed to accept the revised clinical services director position, and May Chandler, a board member, agreed to resign from the board if offered the business manager position. She was prepared to accept that position on a six-month trial at a "salary" of $5 per month plus mileage reimbursement. The job descriptions for the two positions contained overlapping duties that were to be resolved by the two women.

A few board members expressed dissatisfaction with this new staffing arrangement. One believed that Mrs. Traynor should have been appointed administrator, contending that she had never had the chance to prove she could perform that job because she had always performed two roles. Others believed that it was inappropriate to give a volunteer [Mrs. Chandler] authority over paid staff and that it would be difficult for Mrs. Traynor, who previously had full responsibility for the clinic, to report to another person. According to the job descriptions, however, neither position actually reported to the other. Both persons were to attend board meetings and report to the board on separate items.

Mr. Eldridge's view of this situation was:

> All of us on the board—at least those who expressed an opinion on the subject—realized that we were setting up a two-headed monster, an impractical pattern for long-term operation; so all of us, I guess, had doubts about its wisdom. But I could think of no good alternative for moving toward a rational structure with a minimum of discord. I believe the structure was suggested by May, who offered to resign from the board to act as a business manager if we would agree (as we did) to reelect her to the board when it was over. We were able to rationalize this to Angela by pointing out that the job of administrator and chief provider was by then just too much for one person, which was true but only part of the truth.

Although Mrs. Traynor attempted to accept her new position and both women worked to resolve the details of the two positions, Mrs. Traynor was upset by this turn of events. She interpreted the board's decision to create a business manager position and not appoint her to it as a lack of confidence in her abilities and a desire to provoke her resignation. Mrs. Traynor also believed that Mrs. Chandler, under Mr. Eldridge's direction, was documenting her performance to remove her from the position.

In June 1979, after a particularly heated board meeting at which the clinic's utilization problems were discussed once again, Mrs. Traynor resigned. The board accepted her resignation, but retained her as a consultant for two more months. In August, May Chandler resigned as business manager, citing personal reasons. With Mr. Cicero as the clinic nurse practitioner, the board decided to create a part-time administrator position. Between September 1979 and August 1980, two people occupied and subsequently resigned that post. The first part-time administrator was Marlowe Corral, a retired civil service employee with community education and some administrative experience.

Mr. Corral reported that he was hampered from the outset by a lack of board objectives for administering the clinic; the only objectives he could find were in the original grant application. He spent a great deal of his time on accounting matters and claimed that Mr. Eldridge often criticized his results. The board treasurer, an accountant, was asked by the board to assist Mr. Corral with the bookkeeping. The administrator described the board as operational rather than policymaking: "They wanted to know who I have mopping the floors." Mr. Corral resigned in March 1980.

In April, the board hired Betty Gearhart, who had experience in community action program administration, particularly programs for the aging. A new board president was elected in May when Roy Eldridge's term expired, although as past-president he remained on the board and executive committee for one year as an ex officio member. Mrs. Gearhart resigned in August to accept a position closer to her home.

Exhibit Objectives for Cape Meares Health Clinic*

1. To provide within four months of program expansion primary ambulatory health care services to approximately 350 individuals per month. Services will include health screening and assessment, minor illness and injury treatment, health maintenance, rehabilitation, laboratory procedures, electrocardiograms, and information and referrals. Service efforts will continue to be directed toward both the community and the individual.

2. To reduce barriers to care by providing local access to care four days per week after initial expansion and to five days per week after the second year. Health care entities such as stress management, weight control, nutrition planning and other health promotional activities will be made available to the entire population including the presently totally isolated residents of Cape Lookout. Outreach services by boat or van will be available after expansion on the four clinic days and on the weekly community day, bringing beginning services to five days per week and second-year services to six days a week.

3. To provide continuing learning and field experiences for a variety of health care service disciplines including nurses, social workers, and possibly family practice residents. Clinic volunteers will participate in planning their functional roles so that productive use of community talents will continue the valuable contribution to the clinic program. It is anticipated that three to four students will participate each academic quarter.

4. To assure utilization and effectiveness of the health care program, process and product evaluation will be instituted and will include quarterly analysis of utilization surveys and annual studies of program acceptability to consumers. Collaborative research on quality of care will be undertaken with the University of Oregon. Staff for the expanded clinic will include a second nurse practitioner, a professional rural outreach health services worker, a secretary/clerk, a part-time bookkeeper, and a part-time laboratory technician. Expanded services will continue the need for supplementary professional skills of dedicated volunteers. All staff except the second nurse practitioner and the rural health services worker are available and are active in the present clinic program.

*Submitted by Cape Meares Health Clinic in Innovations in Ambulatory Primary Care grant application, 1976.

12
Tehama County Department of Health Services

Tehama County Department of Health Services

In May 1979, Rhonda Dobbs was given an assignment by her supervisor, Dr. Dale Brockman, who was director of the Tehama County Department of Health Services' Division of Public Health. Mrs. Dobbs, who had spent the past four years as director of planning for the Division of Public Health, was to prepare a report on the Brushwood Health Station. Dr. Brockman wanted an analysis of the health station to decide whether to replicate it elsewhere in the county and, if so, whether anything should be done differently. He had selected Mrs. Dobbs for this assignment because she had helped design and implement the Brushwood Health Station.

Mrs. Dobbs knew that the Brushwood Health Station was an unusual entity for a public health department. In fact, she knew that the health department itself was atypical. The changes that had taken place in the county health department beginning in 1970 were the reason the Brushwood Health Station had been formed and at least part of the reason it had succeeded.

To begin her assignment, Mrs. Dobbs thought back over the last 10 years and what had transpired in the county health system and at Brushwood.

Tehama County

Like much of the southwest, Tehama County—the state's most populous county—has been experiencing a population boom. The county population nearly doubled between 1960 and 1975 to 1,246,500. Tehama County's population is concentrated in the San Pablo SMSA, but the county has five other cities with populations over 65,000 and 14 smaller communities of 2,000 to 20,000 residents. A substantial part of the population growth has been in the over-65 age group. The Spanish population is also significant; nearly 15 percent of the county residents are of Spanish heritage.

Geographically, the county is large, covering over 9,000 square miles. A substantial portion of the county is rural with some farmland and large expanses of desert.

A majority of the land in Tehama County—60 percent—is controlled by the federal government through the Forest Service, the Bureau of Indian Affairs or the Department of Defense. The state controls 10 percent and the remaining 30 percent is privately owned. Less than 25 percent of the total land area is subject to state or local taxes.

The Brushwood Region

Brushwood is located 37 miles west of San Pablo. Although it is just beyond the far western edge of the San Pablo SMSA, Brushwood is a remote area because of its low population density and geographic location *(see Figure 1)*. The town of Brushwood has a population of 3,700, but the surrounding rural area, covering 1,850 square miles, brings the total population to 8,000.

In the Brushwood region, over 20 percent of the population is below poverty level, compared to 10 percent countywide. The unemployment rate of 10.6 percent is considerably above the national average. Over one-third of Brushwood's residents are under 15 years of age. The area has somewhat greater proportions of Spanish and black residents than the county as a whole: 22 percent are of Spanish heritage and five percent are black.

History of Tehama County Public Health Services

In the mid-1960s, Tehama County's public health services were limited in scope and largely inaccessible to the indigent population of rural areas. The county health department, located in San Pablo, sponsored categorical programs in public health and preventive medicine, including family planning, prenatal care, immunizations, and screening programs for venereal disease and tuberculosis. But several factors made use of these services difficult. The single-service clinics were offered on different days of the week and in various locations. Travel to the clinics often made them inaccessible. For example, a woman with several children living in the far western part of the county—40 to 50 miles from San Pablo—typically had to visit three different clinics offered on different days of the week to receive medical attention for her family.

While the Tehama County Public Health Department guarded the public health and delivered traditional categorical services, Tehama County General Hospital—also located in San Pablo—provided inpatient services to the indigent sick and injured. Both the health department and the hospital were responsible to the county board of

Figure 1 Tehama County

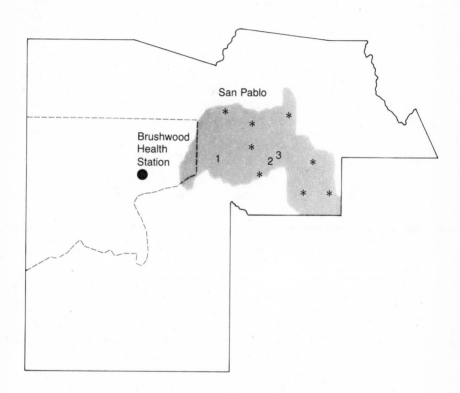

Key

— County boundary
‒ ‒ ‒ Brushwood service area
▨ San Pablo SMSA
1 Saludo Primary Care Center
2 Tehama County Health Department
3 Tehama County General Hospital
∗ Other primary care centers

supervisors, which appointed their governing boards and administrators.

In the late 1960s, the county health department took several steps toward more comprehensive and accessible public health services. First, federal funds were obtained to offer diagnostic and treatment services to certain population groups. One was the south San Pablo children and youth project, and another was the migrant health project. Second, the health department began sending travelling medical teams to isolated areas of the county. Brushwood was one of the areas served by a county medical team. The team—a physician, two nurses, an aide and a clerk—visited each designated area one or two days a week, providing routine medical care and various categorical services.

Financing Public Health Services

Tehama County public health services, which were targeted mainly to the indigent, were financed by the county, state and federal governments. Because of the small county tax base, state and federal sources traditionally were dominant. In the late 1960s, however, several events taking place at the federal and state levels threatened these primary sources for county health funds. First, there was a general decline in federal funding for local health departments. The federal government was providing less support for categorical programs in favor of emphasizing comprehensive care programs. The enactment of Medicare and Medicaid shifted funds from the provision of health care into insurance coverage. However, the state in which Tehama County was located did not participate in Medicaid.

Second, demands on state funds were increasing. The state had been allocating larger amounts of revenue to health departments, including Tehama County, in recent years. Without the influx of federal Medicaid funds, demands on the state budget for health services were greater than ever. The state was in the potential position of having to limit funds for health care or enact Medicaid to obtain federal matching funds.

Tehama County's governing body, the board of supervisors, strongly opposed state participation in the Medicaid program. It was rumored that the county board was behind the state legislature's decision not to participate in Medicaid. One of the supervisors explained the board's opposition to Medicaid this way:

> Other states have implemented a Medicaid program
> and I haven't heard of one that's successful. The
> program seems to foster abuse of the system and
> that's because the control of where the money goes is

no longer with the local people who know what will work best in that area. It seems the federal government is into everything these days and we believe strongly down here that we can take care of our own problems in our own way.

In addition to the desire for independence, the board of supervisors felt that enactment of the Medicaid program would encourage competition in service delivery and thus weaken the role of the health department, which they controlled and which was the single largest health care provider in the state.

As the 1960s drew to an end, the Tehama County board of supervisors was faced with several dilemmas. Access to primary health care continued to be a problem for many indigents in the county. The cost of providing health services was rising but traditional funding sources for the county were being threatened. The county board had to resolve these problems but wanted to do so without giving way to Medicaid participation. The key person to address these issues was the superintendent of the county health department, Russell Sprenger, M.D.

Proposal for an Integrated System

Rising to this challenge, Dr. Sprenger began to plan a cost-effective, accessible health system that would provide a broader range of services and yet not require greater federal funds. He envisioned a countywide system of ambulatory health care centers to provide comprehensive primary care. Secondary and tertiary care would be offered at the Tehama County General Hospital. Dr. Sprenger felt that cost-effectiveness could be achieved systemwide by centralizing the administrative structures, eliminating duplicative services, emphasizing preventive and primary care and streamlining administrative and recordkeeping procedures. If the system worked, the state might be convinced to continue financing the bulk of county public health services without opting for Medicaid participation, and the county board of supervisors might be able to retain its position in health care delivery.

Establishing the Integrated System

Merging the County Health Department and the County Hospital

Dr. Sprenger recognized that some reorganization of the existing services would be necessary. The legal and administrative separation between Tehama County General Hospital and the Tehama County Public Health Department was a barrier to an integrated system. Each had a distinct share of the responsibility for providing health services to the indigent, but there was no policy or administrative coordination between the two structures except that both reported to the county board of supervisors.

Dr. Sprenger and Keith Wilson, the hospital director, worked out a proposal to merge the two structures. In late 1969, they presented the plan to the county board of supervisors. The plan called for an administrative umbrella agency—the Tehama County Department of Health Services (TCDHS)—to oversee both the county hospital and the public health department. Dr. Sprenger felt that centralizing the administration was the first step toward coordinated and efficient services.

Dr. Sprenger's plan seemed to offer a solution to the dilemma faced by the county board of supervisors. After deliberating for several months, the board of supervisors approved the plan in February 1970. They gave Dr. Sprenger the authority to merge the administrative structure of the health department with that of the hospital. During 1971, Dr. Sprenger began by consolidating the personnel divisions and the controller activities of the two organizations.

Two events in 1972 permitted Dr. Sprenger to move to the next phase of his plan—ambulatory primary care centers. In 1972, county residents were voting on a bond issue to construct a new Tehama County General Hospital in San Pablo, one mile from the county health department. Just before the hospital bond issue was released to voters, one county board member—at Dr. Sprenger's behest— persuaded the board to add construction funds for five ambulatory primary care centers to the bond issue. The bond issue for the new hospital and the primary care centers was approved by the voters.

The other event was the state legislature's passage of a law authorizing county boards of health to operate and manage county hospitals. Following passage of this legislation in 1972, the Tehama County board of supervisors consolidated the governing boards of the county health department and the county hospital. The new organization, the Tehama County Department of Health Services, now operated with one board as well as a central administrative structure. It had two divisions: the Hospital Division and the Division of Public Health. Dr. Sprenger was assigned the new post of Assistant County Manager of Health Services to whom both the hospital and public health divisions reported *(Figure 2)*.

In late 1972, Dr. Sprenger enlisted the help of the deputy director at the health department, Dale Brockman, M.D. Dr. Brockman's

Figure 2 Tehama County Department of Health Services

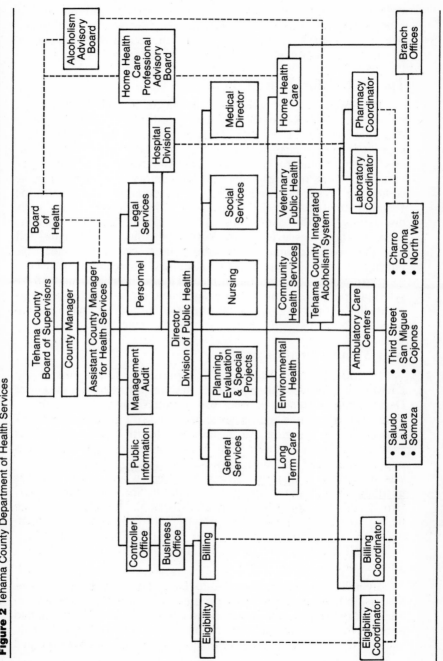

main task was to help set up an organizational and managerial structure for the county health services. He also was to develop key elements of the system, including the patient record system, a budget system and patient eligibility standards for county-paid care.

The Ambulatory Care Committee

Dr. Sprenger felt it was important for the hospital to be involved in making decisions about the system in order to achieve integration and coordination of services. He especially needed the hospital's support of the primary care centers as a referral base for the hospital. Drs. Sprenger and Brockman formed an Ambulatory Care Committee to advise them on organizing the ambulatory care network. The committee was comprised of key representatives from both the Hospital Division and the Division of Public Health. In the early discussions of the Ambulatory Care Committee, the hospital representatives—especially Mr. Wilson, the hospital director—felt that the proposed ambulatory care centers should be under the purview of the hospital division. Although this continued to be a source of contention, the committee did agree on a basic model for a system of peripheral primary care clinics and on cooperative arrangements that should be initiated between the hospital and public health divisions for that system (such as shared pharmacy services).

New Management Strategies

In mid-1973, Dr. Brockman was promoted to director of the Division of Public Health. Soon after that, he proposed that the entire Department of Health Services use a matrix approach to management. He felt that a matrix structure would help resolve conflicts associated with integrating the hospital and health divisions, as well as enable a smoother transition to providing comprehensive services under the merged structure. However, because the hospital director was unconvinced that the matrix approach would work and was unwilling to use it in the hospital division, Dr. Sprenger approved Dr. Brockman's plan only for the health division. One element of the matrix structure called for the primary care centers to use a team management approach. Each center would be managed by three individuals: a clinical director (physician), a nursing supervisor and an administrator.

By mid-1976, the Tehama County Department of Health Services leadership had made significant progress on the new system. Several ambulatory primary care centers were opened. The entire system had adopted the integrated problem-oriented patient records traditionally used by the hospital. Standard principles of practice were developed by the joint medical staffs for use throughout the system. A management information system, a budget system and eligibility standards for patients receiving care in the county delivery system were in place. In addition, the department leadership had conducted orientation and training sessions to introduce all employees to the new organization, management structure and procedures.

In late 1974, Dr. Sprenger retired from his post, satisfied with the progress made in the past several years and satisfied that Dr. Brockman would continue work on the plans for the health division. Jason Howard became the new assistant county manager for health services.

Saludo Primary Care Center

The Saludo Primary Care Center opened in 1972, one of the first of nine in the county's ambulatory care system. The Saludo center—22 miles west of San Pablo—provided a full range of preventive and therapeutic services to a service area population of 10,900. The center was staffed by three physicians, an administrator, seven nurses (a supervisor, three clinic nurses and three field nurses), a medical technologist, pharmacist, social worker and nutritionist. Three of those people comprised the management team for the center. The Saludo center also became the home base for the travelling medical team for the Brushwood area.

In 1975, the team began travelling to Brushwood three days a week to meet a growing demand for services. The team had 2,472 visits by 865 patients during 1975. The majority of the visits (67 percent) were for diagnostic and treatment services rather than for traditional categorical and preventive services. But the travelling medical team was a costly and time-consuming way of providing primary medical care to the indigent and isolated rural population. Moreover, continuity of care was nearly impossible to achieve. Dr. Brockman began looking for an alternative way to serve this population.

The Health Station Concept

In 1975, Dr. Brockman hired Mrs. Dobbs as director of planning for the Division of Public Health. Together they thought of an alternative to the travelling medical teams: health stations that would be an extension of the primary care centers, providing basic primary care in medically underserved, geographically remote areas of the county. The primary care centers would provide more complete outpatient services—such as laboratory and x-ray—for health station patients. Tertiary care, as well as 24-hour emergency care, would be provided by Tehama County General Hospital. Mrs. Dobbs and Dr. Brockman selected Brushwood and the Saludo Primary Care Center to test the health station concept. Mrs. Dobbs was assigned to implement it.

Mrs. Dobbs' preliminary research on the county system and Brushwood indicated the directions she would have to take in designing the health station. First, the health station had to deliver basic medical care but at the same time be a financially feasible element of the county delivery system. Second, the health station had to operate as an extension of the Saludo Primary Care Center but had to reflect the needs of the rural service area.

Mrs. Dobbs completed her plan for the Brushwood Health Station in early 1976 and received Dr. Brockman's approval of it. In the fall, she applied for grant funds from the Hospital Research and Educational Trust's Innovations in Ambulatory Primary Care project to finance it. In June 1977, the Tehama County Department of Health Services was awarded a two-year grant of $84,000 to establish the Brushwood Health Station according to Mrs. Dobbs' plan. To supplement the grant funds and patient charge income,* the county allocated $9,200 to support the Saludo center administrator's salary for time devoted to the health station, equipment costs and office and medical supplies. When the grant ended, the Brushwood Health Station, if continued, would be financed by taxes, as was the rest of the system.

Brushwood Health Station

In June 1977, Maria Castillo was employed by the Tehama County Department of Health Services as family nurse practitioner for the Brushwood Health Station. Mrs. Dobbs' plan was to demonstrate the use of physician extenders—in this case, a family nurse practitioner—in rural primary care settings as both effective and efficient.

A graduate of the state university's family nurse practitioner program and a certified nurse practitioner, Mrs. Castillo had worked as a nurse practitioner in a private physician's office in a rural area and a public health nurse at an Indian community near San Pablo. She was also an assistant professor in nursing education at the state university. Moreover, Mrs. Castillo spoke fluent Spanish.

The Brushwood health station was responsible to the Saludo center's management team—Ann Newport, M.D., medical director, Judy Sharp, R.N., nursing supervisor, and Barry Mills, administrator —and was assigned physician preceptors from the center. David

---

*Mrs. Dobbs estimated that 15 percent of the Brushwood station visits would be billed—two percent to patients and 13 percent to Medicare.

Temple, M.D., was the primary preceptor and Dr. Newport the alternate. An aide, reporting to Mrs. Castillo, was hired to be the health station receptionist, determine patient eligibility for county subsidization and assist in patient care and laboratory work. The health station also had access to the other providers at Saludo, and Saludo's administrator was responsible for training Mrs. Castillo and the aide in administrative and recordkeeping procedures and policies.

During Mrs. Castillo's orientation to the Saludo Primary Care Center and to the county system, she began visiting Brushwood with the travelling medical team. Meanwhile, the 1,400-square-foot storefront building in Brushwood that had been the team's part-time clinic was remodeled.

On October 3, 1977, Mrs. Castillo began treating patients at Brushwood as the sole provider. Estimates were that Brushwood would serve 2,000 patients the first year, 2,600 the second year and 2,950 a year when operating at capacity. When the health station was fully operational, the family nurse practitioner would see 80 patients a week and the physician preceptor 60 patients a week.

The Role of the Nurse Practitioner

The Brushwood Health Station was a model for the Tehama County Department of Health Services not only as a rural care facility but also as a way to utilize the nurse practitioner. Nurse practitioners were new to the patients and to the county health services staff. Success of the Brushwood project depended on acceptance of the family nurse practitioner by both. Consequently, Dr. Brockman and the Saludo center staff made a concerted effort to educate the local community and the TCDHS staff about the role and responsibilities of the family nurse practitioner. Pamphlets describing the family nurse practitioner's activities and her relationship to other staff were distributed. The Saludo management team made presentations about the concept and explained the nurse practitioner and the health station to other primary care center management teams in the county. To gain community acceptance, Mrs. Castillo and Mr. Mills, the Saludo administrator, met with local groups to explain the family nurse practitioner's role at the health station.

Mrs. Castillo recalled her first few months at Brushwood: "Dr. Temple came along and spread the stardust. I would see patients with him and he would say 'this is Maria. This is what she has been doing. She is going to be here when I'm not here.'" Dr. Temple recounted, "When we started out working together, we would see the patient together. I would explain who she was to Spanish patients who had never heard of the concept of a nurse practitioner and just said that she was a special nurse. She came up with that idea. I tried to put in that she was a good provider and she really was."

By January 1978, over 20 protocols had been developed for the independent functioning of the nurse practitioner and a system for medical audits was in place. Dr. Temple audited 100 percent of the records for the first six months and every fourth record thereafter. In addition, he saw each patient for whom Mrs. Castillo requested assistance. Dr. Temple stated, "By this time I felt really comfortable with Maria's decisions and our working relationship. She knows when to refer patients and when she can handle a problem herself."

Brushwood Health Station patients readily accepted the transition from physician to nurse practitioner care. A systemwide audit of the appropriateness of family planning treatment conducted by the Division of Public Health in late 1977 gave another indication of the success of the health station. The audit, evaluating patient records for family planning treatment protocols, showed the quality of care for Brushwood patients to be better than the county average.

Observations on Brushwood

Mrs. Dobbs maintained close contact with the Brushwood Health Station during its formative stage through observation and frequent talks with Mrs. Castillo and others. It was obvious to Mrs. Dobbs that Mrs. Castillo had high regard for the county system. She described it as an "excellent set up" and the network as "the only way to provide the care the patients really need." To Mrs. Castillo, the hospital had "some of the best specialists around." She reported never having a problem in getting information or assistance from the staff.

Mrs. Dobbs attributed the positive relationship between Brushwood and the rest of the system in part to Dr. Brockman's attitude and support: "The whole primary care center and health station concept was really Dr. Brockman's baby. He always kept abreast of any problems that were occurring and most of the time would intervene directly when asked to. He was beginning to turn over more of his primary care center responsibilities to the director of the Ambulatory Care Program, Michael Marciana, partly because he knew he [Brockman] was in line to become the assistant county manager for health services. Mr. Howard, the incumbent, already had announced his intention to leave." Mrs. Dobbs was confident that Mr. Marciana would be an equally strong supporter of the Brushwood Health Station.

Mrs. Castillo's praise of the Tehama County Health Services system was tempered by her frustration with the administrative aspects of her job, which she preferred to minimize in favor of patient care. Paperwork was a problem for Mrs. Castillo, who had only an aide to help her with this responsibility. Furthermore, she felt isolated from the informal communication channels because of the location of the health station (37 miles from the home office), and the fact that the health station was at the "bottom" of the network hierarchy.

Nonetheless, Mrs. Castillo believed that her distance from the Saludo center also had certain advantages. For example, the health station's appointment failure rate was high—often exceeding 25 percent—during the hot summer weather. This was especially true for patients who walked to the clinic. To solve this problem, Mrs. Castillo opened the office at 7 a.m., closed during the heat of the day, and reopened after 3 p.m. when it was cooler. She felt that she would not have been allowed to try an innovation like this in a larger, less flexible operation like the Saludo center.

Mrs. Castillo's major frustration stemmed from the turnover in administrators at the Saludo Primary Care Center that began soon after the Brushwood station opened. Saludo had three administrators in less than two years. These new administrators were unfamiliar with the Brushwood Health Station and with the reporting required by the funding agency; consequently, Mrs. Castillo found herself taking on more administrative duties. She commented, "The Saludo administrators really never knew what was going on out here; they didn't know what the Hospital Research and Educational Trust was, and most times they didn't know what they were supposed to do for us. Every time a new one would come on board I'd have to spend time getting them to realize what I needed from them."

Ken Oliver, who succeeded Mr. Mills and was the administrator at Saludo during 1978, agreed with Mrs. Castillo: "When I came on board, no one explained to me that Brushwood was my responsibility. My understanding was that it was a special project and, while I was supposed to help them out, a lot of other people were looking out for Brushwood too. I had plenty to do just to keep the Saludo center running, and working in the team management structure was a new experience for me that took some adjusting. If there were problems at Brushwood, I would have been glad to help, but everything seemed to be going pretty smoothly."

Mrs. Dobbs was aware that the team management approach at Saludo was not without flaws. She said, "For team management to work, each member must respect the other members and be willing to work cooperatively. You have to learn to fight constructively and if the power between individuals is uneven you've got a real battle. I heard rumors that the management team meetings at Saludo often turned into shouting matches. It's difficult for some physicians to share decision making that's required in this process because they have always functioned independently."

One source of contention among the Saludo staff was the productivity level at the Brushwood Health Station *(Figure 3)*. Dr. Newport, the Saludo medical director, felt that Mrs. Castillo was not scheduling enough patient visits and was working at half capacity. Dr. Newport raised the issue of Mrs. Castillo's productivity at a management team meeting and there was significant disagreement. Dr. Temple, Mrs. Castillo's primary preceptor, also disagreed with Dr. Newport's assessment; he was pleased with her performance and with their working relationship.

The Saludo center also experienced physician turnover that affected Brushwood. When Dr. Newport resigned in July 1978 to relocate with her husband, Dr. Temple was named medical director, although he continued to serve as preceptor for the Brushwood Health Station. Then in early 1979, Dr. Temple was transferred to another county primary care center. The two remaining Saludo physicians alternated serving as Brushwood preceptors. Mrs. Castillo commented, "I had gotten used to working with Dr. Temple and had to make some major adjustments. The patients had gotten used to him too and weren't crazy about change of any sort."

Brushwood's Future

At the start of 1979, there were two key indicators that the Brushwood Health Station was a success. One was the utilization—the station was averaging 400 patient visits a month. The second was the health station's integration into the county health budget as part of the Saludo operation *(Figure 4)*. The county board of supervisors agreed to finance the health station to cover the 70 percent of Brushwood patients who were eligible for county-paid care. This meant that the health station did not have to close with the expiration of the private grant.

Mrs. Dobbs began writing her report to Dr. Brockman. She intended to describe the reasons the model health station had worked and what could have been done differently to make it better and make recommendations on whether and how the model program should be replicated in other areas of the county.

Figure 3 Brushwood Family Nurse Practitioner Activity Data–6/77-5/79

Activity	6/77–5/78	6/78–5/79
Appointments failed (%)	35.5	31.9
Number of patients seen by appointment	1,101	2,058
Walk-ins	605	1,266
Calls to preceptor regarding patients	60	66
Patients referred to preceptor	154	100
Patients seen with preceptor	70	57
*Telephone triage	108	323
†Procedures performed by FNP on-site	529	1,490

*Telephone contact with patients seeking advice.
†Includes immunizations, cultures and lab tests.

Figure 4 Brushwood Health Station Expense Summary–Fiscal Years 1978-1980

	Actual Expenses 6/1/77–5/31/78	Actual Expenses 6/1/78–5/31/79	Adopted Budget 6/1/79–5/31/80
Personnel			
Physician	$10,110	$12,627	$ 6,000
Nurses	12,190	10,548	†
Administration	2,666	5,372	†
*Nurse practitioner	14,007	16,806	18,730
*Health aide	4,488	9,242	11,074
Clerical	729	6,014	†
Other	1,900	-0-	5,200
Fringes	6,683	9,376	4,957
Total	$52,773	$69,985	$45,961
Non-personnel			
*Travel	$ 167	$ 323	$ 510
*Office supplies	236	404	400
*Medical supplies	21,826	27,123	14,700
Equipment	-0-	-0-	1,200
*Rent	2,028	3,120	3,000
Utilities	3,462	2,720	3,255
Telephone	703	1,100	1,390
*Education supplies	-0-	3,113	-0-
Other	4,866	620	50
Total	$33,288	$ 38,523	$24,505
Total Expenses	$86,061	$108,508	$70,466‡

*Grant-supported line items.
†Saludo Primary Care Center contribution.
‡Amount approved by county board of supervisors.

13
Lutheran Hospital

Lutheran Hospital

In 1971, a rudimentary primary care health center opened in Ash Grove, Indiana, to serve a 10-township area with a physician-to-population ratio of 1:6,919. The Ash Grove nurse and homemaker who organized the Ash Grove Family Health Center managed to "borrow" physicians from Monticello, 15 miles away, to staff the part-time venture. This physician arrangement was used until Vern Shelby, M.D., a Monticello physician involved in the Ash Grove Family Health Center and a medical staff member at Lutheran Hospital in Lafayette, Indiana, forged a link between the health center and the hospital's new family practice residency program in 1972. Under this new arrangement, the health center obtained rotating family practice residents and a part-time preceptor from Lafayette and became a full-time, if not fully utilized, operation.

Four years later, in 1976, Lutheran Hospital applied for and received a $146,000, two-year grant from the Hospital Research and Educational Trust (effective April 1, 1977) to convert the Ash Grove Center into a stable and permanent rural practice site for the hospital's growing family practice residency program. Despite these financial resources, the addition of staff at the health center and the closer relationship between Lutheran Hospital and the Ash Grove Family Health Center, the health center was unable to overcome its traditionally low utilization patterns. Nearly two years after the grant was awarded, there were no signs that the health center was capable of remaining viable when the grant funds expired.

Georgia Ottwell, the center's combination nurse and office manager since its inception in 1971, knew that the center's utilization patterns were a problem:

> We just couldn't seem to draw from the permanent population base. From the beginning, the permanent residents of the area never exceeded 60 percent of the total patient load and usually hovered around 50 percent, while the rest of our patients were migrant farm laborers whose care was subsidized by the Indiana Migrant Council. We had no intention of abandoning the migrant population; they were actually our first concern. It's just that we had to pull in many more of the patients who could pay, either directly or through insurers, in order to sustain the health center.

I believe there were two reasons the center couldn't attract a greater percentage of the permanent population: one, the community saw the center as a 'clinic' for the migrant population, and two, there was dissatisfaction with the lack of physician continuity because we had a lot of turnover in physicians over the years followed by residents from Lutheran Hospital who changed every two to three months.

When the hospital stepped in with its plans and resources for revitalizing the health center, I expected to see a big change. But it never really materialized.

Lutheran Hospital

Founded in 1898 by the Lutheran Church, by 1976 Lutheran Hospital was a 500-bed tertiary care facility with a nursing school (one of the first in the state), two residency programs (family practice and pathology) and an ambulatory primary care facility in inner-city Lafayette (operated as a department of the hospital). The hospital also was completing a $20-million expansion that included the addition of a number of ambulatory ancillary services and a facility to house the services.

The hospital's expansion was accompanied by a major reorganization resulting in a management staff with less than two years of tenure in the organization. The new chief executive's long-range plan called for expansion into a broader range of ambulatory care programs, including rural, as one of the diversification goals of the hospital in planning for a sounder financial future. In late 1975, Wade Markle, recently graduated from a midwestern university graduate program in hospital administration, was hired as director of planning and development with responsibility for carrying out the long-range plan.

Mr. Markle was aware of the Family Practice Department's rotating residency experience at the Ash Grove Family Health Center when he learned of the Hospital Research and Educational Trust grant program for demonstrating innovations in ambulatory primary care in medically underserved rural areas. He saw the grant as an opportunity to begin carrying out his charge of expanding the hospital's involvement in ambulatory care. He believed a link between the hospital and the Ash Grove Family Health Center could offer three benefits: a permanent clinical experience for the growing family practice program; a way for the hospital to enter rural primary care and in turn broaden its referral base; and the evolution of a viable and stable health care resource in Ash Grove that could be a prototype for other rural communities.

Recognizing that Dr. Shelby was familiar with the Ash Grove Family Health Center, Mr. Markle discussed his idea with the family practitioner, who was enthusiastic about the opportunity it would afford the still struggling health center. With the backing of the hospital's president, board and family practice residency director, Mr. Markle applied for the grant.

According to the grant application, Lutheran Hospital would channel the grant money into rural ambulatory care initiatives, beginning with the Ash Grove Family Health Center, which would serve as a model for other medically underserved rural communities near the hospital. Two such communities, both with service populations of 2,500 to 3,500 and both with a shortage of physician resources, were identified.

To implement the model at Ash Grove, the family practice residency program, which planned to double its enrollment, would continue to provide the physician resources for the health center. Lutheran Hospital itself "would represent a technical and support service link previously absent at Ash Grove and yet necessary for physicians in primary care practice." As part of this link, the hospital would provide part-time professional support personnel for the center. The grant money itself would be allocated for salaries for the physician and other provider resources at the health center.

When the grant was awarded, Mr. Markle was assigned administrative responsibility for the Ash Grove satellite project.

The Ash Grove Family Health Center

At the time Lutheran Hospital was awarded the grant, the Ash Grove Family Health Center had been in existence about four years. The health center's origin actually could be traced back to 1966, when community members first decided to address the medical needs of the migrant population. While the 9,000 permanent residents of the area could circumvent the local physician shortage by traveling 15 miles to Monticello (where there were five practicing physicians) or 25 miles to Lafayette, that option was not feasible for the 2,000 Chicano farm workers who migrated to the Ash Grove area each April, so they typically went without basic medical care.

The federally-funded Ash Grove Migrant Council and Mrs. Ottwell devised a way to help the migrants. For four years, Mrs. Ottwell drove migrant patients to physicians in Monticello or Lafayette who agreed to treat them; the local migrant council paid the physicians' charges and Mrs. Ottwell's expenses. The local nurse also visited the housing tracts almost daily to provide nursing care.

The transition from these initial efforts for the migrant population to a primary care health center for the entire population was instigated in 1970, when the federal government altered its approach to the funding of migrant health care. Local migrant councils were replaced by state migrant councils, which received federal funds and subcontracted directly with local providers to render services to migrants. Ash Grove had no local providers with whom to employ that approach, but it was eligible for federal subsidies to operate a health care center for treating migrant patients provided that sufficient physician resources could be obtained. To Mrs. Ottwell, this meant that the community did not have to abandon the medical needs of the migrants and at the same time could provide a local resource for the resident population.

Mrs. Ottwell approached two of her closest associates, Rev. Sherman Barclay and Dr. Vern Shelby, with her idea of starting a health care center in Ash Grove. Rev. Barclay, a local pastor, was active in the community and had served on the local migrant council, where he had worked closely with Mrs. Ottwell during the 1960s to arrange medical care for the migrants. Mrs. Ottwell respected his opinion and knowledge of the community and felt he would guide her in the right direction. Mrs. Ottwell also had high regard for Dr. Shelby, whom she described as dynamic and venturesome, enthusiastic about new concepts in family medical care and very involved in community affairs. She had first met the family practitioner while she was a nurse trainee and later became one of his private patients. Dr. Shelby had been on the local migrant council and was one of the few physicians in Monticello who willingly had agreed to devote time from his private practice to treat migrant patients from Ash Grove.

Both Rev. Barclay and Dr. Shelby were enthusiastic about the idea of a local health center. Like Mrs. Ottwell, they believed that the health center should treat not only migrants, and thus qualify for federal funds, but also the entire population. Rev. Barclay and Mrs. Ottwell began eliciting community support for the center. The Atlas Canning Company, which employed migrant farm workers to pick tomatoes each year, pledged a donation for the new health center. Not all of the community members saw a health center as the best solution to the area's medical needs, however. Some, such as pharmacist Andy Gibbons, believed that the best solution was to attract a physician to establish a private practice in the community.

Mrs. Ottwell's next step was to approach the Indiana Migrant Council, the new funding source for migrant health care. The Indiana

Migrant Council was receptive to Mrs. Ottwell's idea, viewing it as a possible prototype for other migrant farm communities in the state. The state council agreed to allocate an annual amount to the health center based on the number of migrant workers treated.*

To house the center, Mrs. Ottwell rented a portion of the Ash Grove pharmacy, owned by Andy Gibbons, and had it renovated. She decided that she could be both nurse and office manager for the health center but needed to find other resources, primarily physicians. She talked to the physicians with whom she had worked since 1966, and several, including Dr. Shelby, agreed to devote a few hours a week to staffing the new health center; some even agreed to donate their time. Mrs. Ottwell hired a part-time receptionist/bookkeeper to complete the staffing complement.

The Ash Grove Family Health Center began providing medical care five afternoons a week in October 1971. The center treated primarily migrant workers, although local publicity emphasized that it was a family health center for everyone.

Family Practice Residents from Lutheran Hospital

Several months after the Ash Grove Family Health Center opened, Dr. Shelby saw the opportunity for a mutually beneficial link between Lutheran Hospital's new family practice residency program and the Ash Grove health center—the hospital could gain a clinical experience site for its residents while the health center would gain providers. In early 1972, through Dr. Shelby's initiative, verbal arrangements were completed with the hospital's Family Practice Department to rotate residents through the Ash Grove Center in three-month cycles.

Because the health center would need a physician preceptor in order to use these physician residents, the hospital's Family Practice Department located a Lafayette-based family practitioner—Dr. Melvin Thompson—who agreed to serve as preceptor on a part-time basis while maintaining his private practice in Lafayette and his affiliation with the residency program. In this manner, the Ash Grove Family Health Center acquired its first "permanent" physician. Although

---

*Under the arrangements between the Indianapolis-based Indiana Migrant Council and the Ash Grove Family Health Center, about $30,000 was allocated to the health center for the provision of migrant health care. The funds could be applied to treatment, ancillary items and overhead expenses. Although Mrs. Ottwell did not know precisely how the Indiana Migrant Council derived the annual allocation, she said that it was somewhat flexible based on her monthly reporting to the state council.

designated the center's medical director, Dr. Thompson only treated patients in conjunction with supervision of the residents and did not direct the center's total patient care activities in the traditional sense.

The Ash Grove Family Health Center's nurse/administrator was glad to have the help of Lutheran Hospital's Family Practice program:

> If the hospital hadn't stepped in, obtaining physician resources would have been our biggest problem, and maybe an unresolvable one. We were really just existing on 'borrowed time' with our initial physician arrangements. The hospital provided residents as well as the physician preceptor, and the cost to us was minimal. The hospital paid their salaries or stipends, and we were obligated to repay the hospital only what we could afford from operating fund excesses, if any. I don't know how else we would have attracted doctors considering our location and financial situation.
>
> At the same time, though, I knew our physician arrangements were perhaps the main reason for the low utilization. The community people didn't like being treated by a different doctor every time they came to the center. That was the case with our borrowed physician resources and it didn't really change with the new resident arrangements.

Mrs. Ottwell also acknowledged that the use of residents presented some practical problems: "We did have to make frequent adjustments in our daily routine. The residents tended to have their own preferences for laboratory procedures and patient appointment scheduling and how they chose to utilize the other center staff. My job was to try to keep things on an even keel and accommodate the physicians at the same time. If a real problem ever arose, I could bring it up to the medical director."

With a physician present every afternoon, the center was able to initiate a full-time schedule. Mrs. Ottwell continued serving as nurse and performing the daily administrative duties, earning a small salary from the migrant funding allocation. Because nursing duties occupied most of her time during regular business hours, Mrs. Ottwell generally performed her administrative tasks in the evening. She also intended to become certified as a nurse practitioner.

The next four years brought little change to the Ash Grove Family Health Center. The expansion of center hours and the addition of residents did little to attract more patients from the permanent population of the service area. When they did utilize the center, it was more often for episodic care than as permanent patients. When Dr. Thompson decided to leave in mid-1976, Lutheran Hospital's Family Practice Department found a replacement from among the program's recent graduates who had set up practice in Lafayette. The new medical director, Dr. Herman Ferris, had practiced at Ash Grove during his residency and was well-liked by the center's patients. Like his predecessor, Dr. Ferris agreed to spend his afternoons at the Ash Grove Family Health Center treating patients and precepting the hospital's residents on rotation there.

Ash Grove Family Health Center as a Satellite

By September 1977, which was midway through the first grant year, Lutheran Hospital had expended slightly over $1,300 of the $146,000 in grant funds designated for the health center. To date, the only visible benefit to the health center was its acquisition of nonphysician professionals: a social worker and a psychologist from the Lafayette Mental Health Center who were employed at Ash Grove part-time through an arrangement between the mental health center and the hospital; and a speech and hearing therapist from the hospital who was assigned to Ash Grove part-time. The therapist's assignment to Ash Grove lasted only one month, however, because of a pressing work load at the hospital. In other areas, the health center was making little or no progress and had even encountered some setbacks.

In the spring of 1977, Dr. Ferris resigned as part-time medical director to open a private practice in Lafayette with the director of the hospital's family practice residency program. Mrs. Ottwell described her feelings about this turn of events: "His leaving was not the main problem because the hospital located a replacement for Dr. Ferris. The part that really upset me was that along with Dr. Ferris went a sizable chunk of our patients—about 150. Most of those who left were permanent residents. They were the ones who were able to go to Lafayette and remain patients of Dr. Ferris. It was a real disaster for the health center."

Another setback occurred when the director of the family practice residency program ordered a change in the rotation shift of the residents. The residents began practicing at Ash Grove in two-month rather than three-month shifts. Patients of the health center who were already dissatisfied with the lack of physician continuity now had even more reason to complain; some simply stopped going to the health center. Health center staff already frustrated by constant adjustments in the daily routine to accommodate the physician residents now had even more cause for frustration.

Mrs. Ottwell asked Mr. Markle to intercede with the Family Practice Department on behalf of the health center. She reported: "He was sympathetic with our plight but said his hands were tied because it was an administrative decision of the family practice residency program." Mrs. Ottwell then turned to the new part-time medical director, Dr. Lozano, who was on the faculty of the residency program. "I figured he had some influence with the program director and could help. He did discuss the problem with the director, Dr. Nesbitt, but to no avail. Dr. Nesbitt refused to alter the resident schedule on the grounds that it would conflict with the requirements and needs of the residency program. He also said something about the changing national accreditation requirements."

Dr. Ed Willow, the health center's part-time psychologist from Lafayette, had a different type of concern:

> Dr. Lozano made no attempt to use my services or those of the social worker in treating patients. We were viewed as a separate entity instead of being integrated into a team approach to delivering care. I discussed this several times with Mrs. Ottwell but nothing happened. I think she simply wanted to steer clear of the medical aspects of the health center's operation, even though she understood what I was saying. I finally decided on a different approach, and Mrs. Ottwell agreed to it. We began holding monthly meetings with all the clinic staff to educate them about psycho-social diagnosis and treatment as an important part of treating the whole patient. Dr. Lozano rarely attended those meetings because of his schedule or other pressing matters. Without Dr. Lozano's support of the concept, it stood little chance of being implemented.

Lutheran Hospital itself was another source of disappointment to Mrs. Ottwell. She now believed that she had misjudged the hospital's commitment to the health center and the results she had anticipated from the association:

> The amount of money the hospital spent from the grant after six months seemed to indicate that the people there weren't committed to following through on their initial plans. As far as I could see, all they had done was arrange to employ some part-time professional staff for the center. Don't misunderstand me—I was very appreciative of the hospital's role in supplying providers. But that apparently wasn't all

that was needed to make the health center come
alive. I think part of the problem was that Wade
Markle was dividing his time between too many tasks.
He was too distant or too distracted to follow through
on his visions of what the health center would become.

As director of planning and development, Mr. Markle saw the
health center as a small but important part of his job. His time on the
project was devoted primarily to interacting with and reporting to the
grant agency. He intentionally tried to restrict his involvement in the
health center's operation. Most of his contacts with Ash Grove were
via telephone. If needed, he could contact the medical director, Dr.
Lozano, while he was on his rounds at the hospital.

In the fall of 1977, Mr. Markle was promoted to vice-president for
ambulatory services. He also was negotiating with a community group
in Brookston to establish a second clinic there, patterned after Ash
Grove, by February 1978. According to Mr. Markle, his new post,
while encompassing many hospital programs, would allow him more
time to concentrate on the Ash Grove and Brookston clinics.

Mrs. Ottwell detected no change in Mr. Markle's attention to Ash
Grove despite his new position and his contention that it would allow
him more time for the health center. She did not believe that his low
profile with the center was intentional, however: "My impression from
Dr. Lozano and Dr. Shelby, both of whom knew a lot more about the
hospital than I did, was that Mr. Markle was subject to the priorities
and whims of the hospital. With his other responsibilities and the
reorganization at the hospital, he just didn't have the energy to devote
to us."

A Community Advisory Board

As 1977 turned into 1978, Mrs. Ottwell had a growing fear that the
health center was failing. Her reliance on the hospital and the medical
director had so far been disappointing, so she decided to try the only
other approach she could think of that might work—a community
advisory board. During the health center's earliest years, there had
been a community advisory board, but internal dissension over the
best approach to health care services for the community and the onset
of the hospital's involvement through the residency program had
precipitated the board's dissolution.

Mrs. Ottwell's hope was that a community advisory board could
somehow address the health center's biggest problem—utilization.
She contacted a number of people, including many who had been on

the original advisory board, to attend a meeting in February 1978 at the church. Mrs. Ottwell stated, "I didn't know how the hospital would react to this idea but decided to take a gamble. As it turned out, Mr. Markle didn't oppose it and even agreed to participate on the board."

Mr. Markle agreed to the advisory board concept for a variety of reasons: "I firmly believed that the health center should assume whatever form would work best under the particular circumstances. I knew that the health center had to become an integral part of the service area to have any hope of retaining good health professionals. If the health center failed, the community would lose and so would the hospital. A final factor was that the grant agency had been pushing the idea for some time based on positive experiences of other health centers in similar circumstances."

The meeting, which was attended by about 15 people, turned into an emotionally-charged forum where many issues surrounding the health center were raised by both community representatives and center staff. According to Rev. Barclay, the community avoided the health center because of its physicians: "People don't feel comfortable or confident in the care they're receiving when a new doctor sees them every time. And some have told me they don't completely trust the residents because they're students and not full-fledged doctors." Dr. Lozano admitted that people may harbor those feelings, but called them groundless: "All that's needed is an education process. People have to overcome the country doctor syndrome—it's a thing of the past. These residents know the latest techniques in medical care. The patients are getting the best care possible and I'm here to make sure of that."

Dr. Willow and the center's bookkeeper/receptionist presented another side of the issue, discussing the internal problems caused by transient physicians. Dr. Willow even believed that the physicians had little loyalty to the center. Dr. Lozano refuted that claim. "Although I can't really speak for those who preceded me in this post," Dr. Lozano said, "I have strived to do my best for the health center and its patients and to cultivate the same attitude in the residents who come here. We have established good rapport with the patients and particularly the migrants, who have a language barrier. When I took this job, I made it clear that I would eventually be relocating to another part of the country, but that in no way has affected my dedication to the center."

Pharmacist Andy Gibbons believed that the health center's image as a clinic for migrants was the key factor in deterring the permanent residents. He said permanent residents resented the fact that they had to wait for appointments and for treatment while migrants simply walked in without an appointment and were treated right away. Both Dr. Lozano and Mrs. Ottwell responded in defense of the migrants: "They can't plan their work day in advance or take time off from their job to use the health center as easily as other people can. We have to be sensitive to that." Dr. Lozano explained that the migrants had the opposite complaint—they had to take time off from work if they wanted to receive treatment. The health center had once instituted evening hours for that reason but abandoned them due to difficulties in scheduling providers and a poor response from consumers.

A recent letter to the local newspaper was read at the meeting. In it, a woman complained that she had been refused emergency treatment at the health center when her regular physician was not available. Mrs. Ottwell pointed to the letter as a prime illustration of how the community viewed the health center: "It's just somewhere to go when their regular physicians are unavailable." Looking around the room, Mrs. Ottwell observed that most of those present were not regular patients of the health center for that very reason.

There was unanimous agreement that the center's facility was also a major problem. It was cramped, offered little patient privacy and precluded any possibility of service expansion. (Mr. Markle neglected to bring up the fact that, even before the grant was awarded to the hospital, the grant agency had pointed out to him that the health center lacked adequate space for the service objectives stated in the grant application. He reportedly had not brought up the matter because of building owner Gibbons' adamant position that the facility was adequate for a physician's office.)

Before the meeting ended, plans were made to set up a community advisory board to address the health center's problems and the broader issue of health care resources for the community. Thirteen members, including officers, were elected to the advisory board in April 1978. Among them were Dr. Lozano and Mrs. Ottwell from the health center, Mr. Markle and an accountant from the hospital, Rev. Barclay, Dr. Shelby and Grady Lewis, the Atlas company's plant manager.

Agreeing that the health center should continue to serve both permanent residents and migrants, the advisory board adopted a two-tier approach to the community's health care needs. The short-term goal was to foster greater community utilization of the center by (1) improving physician continuity through a better resident rotation schedule, (2) promoting the health center and (3) enlarging the facility. The long-term goal was to recruit a permanent physician who would reside in the service area.

As 1978 progressed, the community advisory board succeeded in some areas but was met with disappointment in others. Mr. Gibbons refused to allow any expansion to the building. An application for Rural Health Initiative funds was tabled by the regional federal office because funds were unavailable at the time. The board learned from Mr. Markle that its composition did not meet federal requirements for consumer representation under the migrant aid program. Attempts to recruit a permanent physician were unsuccessful. Newspaper articles, a new brochure, a larger sign for the center and an open house did little to improve its utilization.

At the board's final meeting of 1978, Rev. Barclay proposed that the Ash Grove Family Health Center file for status as a nonprofit community corporation governed by a board of directors with a consumer majority. The resolution passed unanimously. At the same meeting, Mr. Markle presented a management contract offer from the hospital *(Exhibit 1)*. It was rejected in favor of appointing Mrs. Ottwell full-time administrator, although she still would need to devote some time to nursing activities. With no alternative in sight for physician resources, the board decided to continue using Lutheran Hospital residents. Letters of agreement were drawn up between the hospital on behalf of its family practice residency program and the health center *(Exhibits 2 and 3)*. While they made provision for evening coverage at the health center, the rotation schedule remained basically unchanged.

As 1979 began, the Ash Grove Family Health Center advisory board was convinced that some positive steps had been taken toward self-reliance. Still eluding the board, however, were solutions to the two main barriers in the way of achieving that self-reliance: physicians and patients.

Exhibit 1 Lutheran Hospital Management Contract Proposal to the Ash Grove Family
Health Center Board of Directors

Lutheran Hospital of Lafayette proposes to offer certain management services as
described below.

1. Preparation of a long range plan, including an analysis of the present situation,
and recommendations regarding future activities and programs, staff, facilities,
and equipment.

2. Assistance in financial and accounting procedures and systems.

3. Assistance in personnel policies and systems including wage and salary,
training, and organization.

4. Assistance in purchasing policies and procedures.

5. Provision of management training for the Family Health Center administration.

6. Assistance in general administrative areas regarding organization, operation,
and development of the Family Health Center.

Management Arrangement

1. An administrative person acceptable to the Board would be provided by the
Lutheran Hospital.

2. This person would spend one day per week consulting at the Ash Grove Family
Health Center and also report at Board meetings.

3. Georgia Ottwell would spend one day per week at Lutheran Hospital in
management training and working under the guidance of the assigned administrative person who would coordinate consultation from other hospital staff.

4. This arrangement would continue for one year unless terminated by the Board
of Directors.

5. The management contract service time would represent .4 FTE at $12,000 per
year.

Exhibit 2 Letter of Agreement: Daytime Physician Services

Lutheran Hospital of Lafayette through its Family Practice Residency Program agrees to provide physician services to staff the Ash Grove Family Health Center during regular afternoon office hours at least four afternoons weekly. Additionally, inpatient and emergency care at Lutheran Hospital will be provided to patients of the Ash Grove Family Health Center. In return for these services, the Ash Grove Family Health Center agrees to reimburse Lutheran Hospital of Lafayette $20.00 per hour of physician time spent at the Ash Grove Family Health Center plus a mileage allowance of $.17 per mile. The hourly fee shall be paid directly to Lutheran Hospital and the mileage fee shall be paid directly to the physician. As Lutheran Hospital of Lafayette will be providing malpractice coverage for the physician, it agrees to hold the Ash Grove Family Health Center harmless and indemnified from the acts or omissions of the physician.

The term of this agreement shall be from December 15, 1978, to December 14, 1979.

Agreed:

_____

Lutheran Hospital

_____

Ash Grove Family Health Center

_____

Exhibit 3 Letter of Agreement: Evening Physician Services

Lutheran Hospital of Lafayette agrees to provide licensed physician services to staff evening clinics sponsored by the Ash Grove Family Health Center. In return for these services, the Ash Grove Family Health Center agrees to reimburse Lutheran Hospital $25.00 per hour of physician service provided, plus mileage @ $.17 per mile if exclusive of other mileage reimbursement agreements. As Lutheran Hospital of Lafayette will be providing malpractice coverage for the physician, it agrees to hold the Ash Grove Family Health Center harmless and indemnified for the acts or omissions of the physician.

The term of this agreement shall be from December 15, 1978, to December 14, 1979.

Agreed:

_____

Lutheran Hospital

_____

Ash Grove Family Health Center

_____